MYSTICAL
D·I·E·T·S

Consumer Health Library®
Series Editor: Stephen Barrett, M.D.
Technical Editor: Manfred Kroger, Ph.D.

Other titles in this series:

MYSTICAL

D✷I✷E✷T✷S

Paranormal,

Spiritual,

and Occult

Nutrition

Practices

JACK RASO, M.S., R.D.

EDITED BY STEPHEN BARRETT, M.D.

Prometheus Books • Buffalo, New York

6/95

Published in 1993 by Prometheus Books.

Mystical Diets: Paranormal, Spiritual, and Occult Nutrition Practices.
Copyright © 1993 by Jack Raso. All rights reserved. No part of this
publication may be reproduced, stored in a retrieval system, or transmitted
in any form by any means, electronic, mechanical, photocopying, record-
ing, or otherwise, without prior permission of the publisher, except in the
case of brief quotations embodied in critical articles or reviews. Inquiries
should be addressed to Prometheus Books, 59 John Glenn Drive, Buffalo,
NY 14228-2197, 716-691-0133 (FAX: 716-691-0137).

97   96   95   94   93   5   4   3   2   1

Library of Congress Cataloging-in-Publication Data

Raso, Jack
    Mystical diets: paranormal, spiritual, and occult nutrition
practices / by Jack Raso.
    p.   cm.   Consumer Health Library
Includes biographical references and index.
ISBN 0-87975-761-2 (acid-free, cloth)
    1. Diet therapy. 2. Nutrition. 3. Alternative medicine. 4. New Age
Movement.   I. Barrett, Stephen, 1933–   . II. Title.   III, Series.
RM217.R33 1992
613.2'6—dc20

                                                92–40828
                                                CIP

Printed in the United States on acid-free paper.

For my mother, Josephine Raso,
and my aunt and uncle,
Pauline and Michael Pendola

About the Author

Jack Raso is a registered dietitian who lives in New York City, where he was born and raised. A humanities major from 1972 to 1974, Mr. Raso attended three vocational schools before returning to college in 1981. In 1985, he graduated summa cum laude from Pratt Institute in Brooklyn with a B.S. degree in nutrition and dietetics. Later that year, he was granted a teaching fellowship at Long Island University, where he pursued an M.S. degree in health science. Mr. Raso has taught at the undergraduate and graduate levels, has lectured in a variety of settings, and since early 1991 has been a contributing editor of *Nutrition Forum* newsletter. A member of the National Council Against Health Fraud, he is collaborating on an encyclopedia of "paranormal healing" and expects to pursue a doctorate in health services.

About the Editor

Stephen Barrett, M.D., who practices psychiatry in Allentown, Pennsylvania, is a nationally renowned author, editor, and consumer advocate. An expert in medical communications, he edits *Nutrition Forum* newsletter and is medical editor of Prometheus Books. He is a board member of the National Council Against Health Fraud and chairs the council's Task Force on Victim Redress. His thirty-two books include: *Vitamins and "Health" Foods: The Great American Hustle; Health Schemes, Scams, and Frauds; Reader's Guide to "Alternative" Health Methods;* and the college textbook *Consumer Health: A Guide to Intelligent Decisions.* In 1984 he won the FDA Commissioner's Special Citation Award for Public Service in fighting nutrition quackery. In 1987 he began teaching health education at The Pennsylvania State University.

Contents

Acknowledgments

The following persons facilitated the writing of this book in miscellaneous ways: providing transportation, information, technical assistance, moral support, and/or incitement. Artist Yasutaka Ishimaru was my leading inspiration. Social worker Varghese Kodiyan, M.A., M.S.W. C.S.W., medical librarian Inna Lipnitsky, M.S.L.I.S., and computer consultant Young K. Rick were extraordinarily supportive. I also thank Harry Chung and Yelena Vasilyeva, M.S.

During the editing process, I was greatly helped by: Manfred Kroger, Ph.D., Professor of Food Science, The Pennsylvania State University (technical editing); Steven L. Mitchell, editorial director, Prometheus Books (project manager); and Michael Botts, Esq., specialist in health law, Kansas City, Missouri (legal review).

Finally, I would like to pay tribute to my editor, Stephen Barrett, M.D., who tolerantly, lighthandedly, almost imperceptibly guided this one-time "alternative" healthcare admirer on the path to discerning skepticism.

1

From Believer to Skeptic: My Personal Odyssey

Paranormal Nutrition

Despite its title, this book is not as concerned with diets, "mystical" or other, as it is with the metaphysical beliefs that have enraptured—at no small expense—dieters, food faddists, "immortalists," seekers of "high-level" wellness, and undiscerning nutrition buffs. Over the past quarter-century, I have evolved from a believer into a skeptic.

In the process, I took overdoses of vitamins; worked in three "health food" stores; read hundreds of scientific and unscientific nutrition publications; consulted "alternative" practitioners as a patient; acquired a baccalaureate in scientific nutrition and a master of science degree in health science and exercise physiology; attended a dozen "alternative" healthcare courses and conferences; applied to eight unconventional programs and a graduate program in Christian theology; and examined Anthroposophy, applied kinesiology, Ayurveda, the Edgar Cayce tradition, chiropractic, Gerson therapy, herbalism, homeopathy, macrobiotics, multilevel marketing, nutripathy, Theosophy, trance channeling, and other "New Age" and religious beliefs and practices.

This book represents a catharsis and an attempt to share what I have learned.

In the field of human nutrition and dietetics, the term "normal nutrition" refers to nutritional considerations for health maintenance, as distinct from therapeutic nutrition, a form of medical treatment. "Paranormal nutrition" is an umbrella term I have coined for unscientific nutrition-

1

related beliefs, practices, and systems—particularly those with supernatural premises and a cult-like ambiance. Such systems have been proposed for the recovery, preservation, or improvement of health.

My work on this book has elicited puzzlement from acquaintances and colleagues alike. Just how does one become a "specialist" in paranormal nutrition?

Paranormal Dreamin'

My odyssey began during childhood in an environment conducive to magical thinking. Thirteen years of Roman Catholic schooling constituted the seedbed for my once unlimited credulity. Parochial school conditioned me to take for granted such ideas as the presence of Christ in the Eucharistic bread. Another teaching, more insidious, held that one would receive anything requested from "God the Father" in the name of Jesus Christ. In high school, with the progressive modernization of the Roman Catholic Mass and its consequent demystification, I rebelled, perusing all manner of Western occult literature antithetical to Christianity, including Anton Szandor LaVey's *Satanic Bible*. LaVey's message was bizarrely similar to the Christian teaching closest to my heart, in essence: "Ask according to ritual, and you shall receive." After my graduation from high school in 1972, a friend lent me a small book on reincarnation that, to my mind, legitimized the occult.

I thus made my transition from mainstream paranormal believing to unbridled, anti-establishment paranormal believing. It was perhaps my unconventionality that provoked the mother of an erstwhile friend to take me to a faith-healing session, wherein I simulated the "gift of tongues." But I was by no means healed.

Less than two years after graduation, when I was nineteen, I performed a ritual in my basement that seemed to yield the intended result. The ritual was described in a testimonial-laden book I had ordered by mail. In the ritual, I visualized receiving a particular phone call, and the call came only moments afterward. This occurrence, which I now realize was utterly insignificant statistically, helped keep me comfortably undecided about the reality of supernatural phenomena.

My uncritical thinking allowed me to engage in such activities as Buddhist chanting, which I performed both privately and at local meetings of a sect named Nichiren Shoshu of America. There I was taught that by chanting mystical words repeatedly—especially "*Nam myoho renge kyo*" and preferably in front of a sacred scroll—I could accomplish whatever I desired. In later years, my supernatural bent was reinforced by self-help books, such as Claude Bristol's *The Magic of Believing*, that advocate quasi-religious rituals.

Supplement Junkie

During my early twenties, I gradually awakened to the finitude of youth and life and grew obsessed with preserving myself for an undefined breakthrough that would somehow descend upon me. I was a student at a vocational school, working part-time in a library, when I became interested in dermatology. My interest in nutrition began when I read *The Natural Way to Super Beauty* (1974), which processes the recommendations of such "eminent figures in nutrition and medicine" as Robert Atkins, Linda Clark, Adelle Davis, Carlton Fredericks, Frances Moore Lappe (*Diet for a Small Planet*), and Maxwell Stillman (*The Doctor's Quick Weight Loss Diet*). Further reading prompted my first visit to a "health food" store, where I was awed by the array of esoteric supplements preceded by paperback displays. I selected a book on vitamin E and afterward bought several bottles of chewable vitamin supplements at a discount store. Then I read a paperback on how to retard the aging process with nutritional supplements. It did not take long for me to become immersed in the popular nutrition literature.

Later I followed a low-carbohydrate "health food" diet and dabbled in "food combining" à la Natural Hygiene. Supplementation turned from a hobby of sorts into an addictive passion for supplements, "health foods," nutrition-related books, and even photocopies of nutrition-related articles. I was underweight and weak. My skin was pallid, dry, and flaky, and I had dandruff and a dry, itchy scalp. It was not unusual for my appearance to evoke inquiries regarding my health. Not uncommonly, nausea, stomach-aches, and diarrhea would follow my ingestion of supplements, and I became used to finding them virtually intact in my stool. A urinalysis arranged by a concerned teacher revealed ketonuria, a sign of semistarvation.

Between 1979 and 1981, my health apparently improved with an unrestricted high-fat diet and regular exercise. I followed the recommen-dation in a book on bodybuilding to drink half-and-half, until I read a newspaper article by Nathan Pritikin deprecating intake of fats across the board. Without a prescription, I procured Gerovital H3 (GH3), a procaine preparation claimed to have anti-aging effects, from a "health food" store.

Not infrequently, I would swallow upwards of seventy-five pills and capsules daily, plus many assorted herbal extracts—despite nausea, vomiting, headaches, cramps, diarrhea, and rashes. I actually developed calluses on my left hand from opening and securely closing dozens of supplement bottles daily.

The Trichologist Was Out

I did read such critical books as *The Health Robbers* (1980) and *Nutrition Cultism: Facts and Fictions* (1981), whose reports of the seamy side of the health marketplace gave me pause. But my elaborate supplementation regimen, though adjustable, was a fixture because it made me a special mortal. To me, it was a badge, if not a guarantee, of health and longevity. Furthermore, the critical books I came across were far outnumbered by uncritical books and articles that supported what I was doing.

The books and magazines sold in the "health food" stores that I haunted advocated "alternative" medicine, which appealed to me mainly because of its emphasis on "harmless" nutritional methods with which I was familiar. I saw an ad for a directory of "nutrition-minded" physicians and dentists, ordered it, and made an appointment with one of the dentists. My visit with him differed from my previous dental care in four ways. First, I was given a diet history form to complete at home. Second, one of his staff offered me a "high-protein" milk shake. Third, I was given two calcium tablets, which, I was told, would protect me against the effects of the dental x-rays. Last, the dentist advised me in no uncertain terms to have my mercury-amalgam fillings removed and have my teeth capped with gold inlays. I did not follow his counsel, because it struck me as odd to have to go to so much trouble only to wind up with less tooth enamel.

Unhappy over the thinning of my hair at the crown, I also attempted to consult a "trichologist" (nonmedical hair "specialist") whose ad I'd seen in a newspaper. I arrived on time for my appointment, but was told he was not scheduled for that location (a chiropractic facility) on that day. Instead, I was seen by a chiropractor who offered dietary assessment and counseling. Two different diagrams of a hair shaft and follicle hung on the wall: one allegedly representing the potential for normal hair growth, the other representing male-pattern baldness. The chiropractor plucked a few of the thinner hairs from my head, projected a microscopic view of them onto a screen, pronounced them normal, and assured me (erroneously) that the thinning of my hair was not due to male-pattern baldness and could thus be corrected. He sold me a plastic shampoo brush and three unlabeled hair-care products—said to be a shampoo, a conditioner, and a grooming lotion—all for "just" $125. He also prescribed treatment involving scalp massage, ultraviolet irradiation, and a contrivance that emitted an herbal mist—which was administered in his office by a staff member with long fingernails. I refused to be irradiated, threw out the products within a week, and never returned.

In 1981, my fascination with nutrition, my perplexity, and my longing for a career consistent with my interests emboldened me to undertake formal study of the subject. Over the years I spent as an undergraduate nutrition major, I would typically consume daily over 7,500 mg of vitamin C, more than 2,500 IU of vitamin E, 750 mg of the artificial food preservative BHT, pyridoxal-5-phosphate (the cofactor form of vitamin B_6), germanium, lithium orotate, alfalfa, choline, inositol, RNA, and so forth. I subscribed to *Anti-Aging News* (a newsletter for "immortalists" and so-called life-extenders), enthusiastically read *Recalled By Life* (a book about a doctor with cancer who turned to macrobiotics), produced my own "version" of Gerovital by purchasing the anesthetic procaine hydrochloride at a drug-paraphernalia shop and encapsulating it, sweetened my cereal with inositol, and bought my supplements wholesale.

"Nutrition Consultant" at GNC

When I was an undergraduate, I was employed part-time at three "health food" stores. One was independent and two were operated by General Nutrition Corporation (GNC). At GNC, I passed a simple take-home exam and thus became a "nutrition consultant," as indicated on my name badge. Salespeople were expected to accost every potential customer and recite a sales pitch for a chewable vitamin C supplement. Compliance was monitored via "plainclothes" collaborators who "shopped" us under the direction of area supervisors. I became acting assistant manager at GNC. Commissions provided both managers and salespersons with the incentive to sell. My manager made public my majoring in nutrition and referred to me as "the professor." She represented herself as a registered nurse to area supervisors, salespersons, and customers. Despite the many nutritional products in the store marketed to dieters or claimed in the "health food" literature to facilitate weight loss, this manager repeatedly bemoaned the enduring fact of her obesity. I found working in all three of these stores demeaning, because of the pressure to sell useless products to unwise

people and the near-total disregard for nutritional science. At the independent health-food store, an herbalist, not employed by the store, saw clients
by appointment and prescribed herbal preparations sold there. Aware of
my scientific training, he seemed bothered by my presence.

From Yoga to Crystals

During the 1980s, I also enrolled in courses in hatha yoga and meditation
at the Himalayan Institute of New York, which shares its site with an
affiliated "metaphysical" bookstore called East West Books. The meditation instructor told us he had met "breatharians" in the Himalayas—yogis
who subsist virtually on air alone by extracting nitrogen from it. I didn't
believe him and decided I would postpone seeking answers to metaphysical questions at least until graduation. Yet, germinating within me was a
desire to formulate a coherent, perennial philosophy of nutrition. Skepticism was not taught at college, and I had little understanding of it. Thus I
often resorted to instinct when reading health-related publications. Michio
Kushi's *Book of Macrobiotics*, which I bought at the Himalayan Institute's
bookstore, did not ring true. A book on Rudolf Steiner's nutritional views
struck me as so outdated I returned it the next day for a refund. The seeds
of my eventual disillusionment had been planted.

En route to becoming a registered dietitian, I attended graduate
school. By the time I earned my master's degree in health science in 1987,
I was taking only a handful of supplements daily and had weeded my small
library of nearly all uncritical popular nutrition literature (much to my
present regret, since I am now writing about it). But a year later I suffered
a personal loss that left me confronting what I termed "spiritual bank-
ruptcy." Prayers hailing from the time of my religious instruction proved
a waste of time. Resolute in my quest, I began frequenting East West
Books and several other metaphysical bookstores. I found inspiration in
UFO "abductionist" Whitley Strieber's *Communion*. I bought crystals,
even though I had only the vaguest notion about why or how they
supposedly should be used. And I blindly pursued an intimate relationship
with a disarming self-styled witch and Buddhist who practiced *pranayama*
daily, spoke absorbingly of "World Teachers" and the fabled *Necronomicon*,
and could supposedly appraise an individual's "aura" even via a photograph. The articulateness and seeming erudition of this occultist were such
that I half-believed.

Reality Dawns

At this juncture, my winding road to skepticism entered the "twilight zone" of nutrition and dietetics. During my sojourn there, I seem to have experienced a state of mind termed the "Dark Night of the Soul" in the mystical literature—a stage of spiritual development characterized by depression, disbelief, uncertainty, and self-doubt, which, typically, directly precedes a breakthrough to fresh understanding. Such a breakthrough did in fact occur, gradually—perhaps the selfsame breakthrough for which I had sought to preserve myself, but could not define, in my relative youth. It was a breakthrough to qualified, constructive skepticism, critical thinking, and self-understanding.

What caused this breakthrough? Opportunities to write for *Nutrition Forum*, a unique newsletter published and edited by Stephen Barrett, M.D., spurred me to delve into macrobiotics, Natural Hygiene, the Edgar Cayce tradition, "complementary" medicine, the Matol movement, and herbalism. Macrobiotics represents my intellectual watershed, for I became a skeptic as a result of attending a discomfiting seminar held at the Kushi Institute (the macrobiotic "Vatican") in mid-1989. My experiences there are described in Chapter 3. Since then, I have spent thousands of dollars and many sleepless nights trying to fathom philosophical questions, "New Age" beliefs and trends, and "alternative" health care. In 1991, I concluded that many "alternative" healthcare systems were religions of a sort, and I devised this book.

In the next chapter, I try to convey a broad but practical understanding of "alternative" health care and its philosophical foundations. Subsequent chapters deal with specific types.

2

The "Holistic" Bandwagon: Defective Parts and a Supernatural Chassis

What Is "Alternative" Medicine?

There is a thread that runs through most of the "healing" systems described in this book: In many cases, proponents claim that ailments can be cured, modified, or prevented by stimulating, directing, and/or altering the body's "vital force" or "healing power," which goes by many names. Such "treatment" is not based on an understanding of pathology and biochemistry accrued through the scientific method, but on anecdotes, testimonials, mythology, and religious thinking. Unleashing "healing energy" is supposed, for example, to improve immune function and thus increase resistance to disease.

Such nonscientific approaches are lumped under a variety of ambiguous names: usually with the word "medicine" or "healing" preceded by *alternative*, *complementary*, *extentional*, *fringe*, *holistic* (or *wholistic*), *innovative*, *New Age*, *nontraditional*, *unconventional*, or *unorthodox*. In the January 2, 1992 *New England Journal of Medicine*, Drs. Raymond H. Murray and Arthur J. Rubel write:

Alternative practices represent a hodgepodge of beliefs and treatments. Many are well known, others are exotic and mysterious, and some are dangerous. They are based on no common or consistent ideology, theory of illness, or treatment. They derive from a wide variety of sources: ethnic and folk traditions, mainstream medical practices, established religions or semireligious cults, philosophies or metaphysical movements, and health-and-

9

wellness groups exploiting the growing rebellion against technology and the perceived impersonalization of medical care.

Proponents of "alternative" methods seldom criticize their own or other "alternative" systems. Despite the disparity of their beliefs, advocates of particular systems rarely argue or compete with one another; in league against scientific health care, they tend to view one another as complementary. While "alternative" medicine tends to be all-accommodating despite sectarian differences, scientific medicine is self-critical and coherent. Self-criticism is essential for scientific progress, but it also provides convenient targets for "alternative" promoters to attack in "competing" for public support.

Karl Sabbagh illustrates the theoretical abyss of fringe medicine in the Winter 1985-86 issue of *Skeptical Inquirer*:

> Is kidney disease rooted in the bottom sector of the iris [per iridology] or the center of the sole of the foot [per foot reflexology], or several different [acupuncture] points in the ear or perhaps at the lower end of this complex set of [alleged] energy zones?

Despite all this, a few mishaps, misunderstandings, or bad experiences can disanchor an individual from scientific health care. (The feeling that a doctor has been too brusque regarding psychosomatic symptoms is an oft-quoted example.) Then a few popular books or magazines can disrudder the individual, leaving him to float from one "alternative" system to another.

May the (Vital) Force Be with You!

Although dissimilar in veneer, "alternative" healing systems share a rhetoric involving a dubious interlocking triad of vitalism, mind-body interactionism (in "holistic" disguise), and empiricism.

Discussions affirming the existence of a "vital force" are now rare in scientific settings, but are not unheard of. For example, as late as 1973, a "scientific" article was published in Japan, in which a former director of a medical school's physiology department wrote: "A certain force, which is contained in a living body, is making the organs of animal body work during its whole life." This is the crux of vitalism. "Vitalism" refers to the doctrine or proposition that a unique form of energy, neither chemical nor mechanical, distinguishes living from nonliving things. In *Planet Medi-*

cine (1987), "alternative" medicine proponent Richard Grossinger, Ph.D., defines vitalism as

> at once, a science, a religious philosophy, and a doctrine which radically alters all other theories of matter and being. It states that life is unique, that it possesses properties in some manner above and beyond its physics and chemistry. In some versions, even inanimate matter contains a slumbering vital force that can be aroused.

Traceable to the philosopher Aristotle (384–322 B.C.E.) and to Galen (130–200 C.E.), the father of medicine, the "vital force" hypothesis has not had any real scientific importance since the late eighteenth century. But the term survives in informal speech and represents a major difference between the scientific and nonscientific approaches to biology and physiology. A core of vitalism marks many "alternative" healing systems as religious rather than scientific in nature. Macrobiotics refers to this alleged "vital principle" as *Ch' i* or *ki,* Natural Hygiene as "essence" or "life force," the Edgar Cayce tradition as the spirit or soul, Ayurvedic medicine as *prana,* and fundamentalist chiropractors as "Innate Intelligence." While the terms are not always interchangeable, they certainly point to the same theme. The term "vital principle," proposed in the eighteenth century, is just a fancy way of saying "soul."

Both Aristotle and Galen, and the alchemists as well, believed that food, too, contained a "basic vital element" or life-sustaining "essence." In the nineteenth century, it was commonly believed that all foods contained a single "universal element" that sustained life; consequently, quantity was emphasized rather than quality. In 1974, in the *Journal of the American Medical Association*, "quackbuster" Thomas H. Jukes, Ph.D., D.Sc., cited vitalism in its broader sense as responsible for the preference of "health food" advocates for fertilized eggs and "natural" fertilizers and vitamins.

Many such advocates hold that there is something in living things that cannot be measured by modern scientific instruments. In 1971, a few months after the death of J.I. Rodale, *Prevention* magazine published a glowing tribute. Calling him the "father of natural food supplements," the editor wrote:

> It took the simple vision of J.I. Rodale to see that synthetic vitamin C being sold ... from thousands of drugstores was not alive and had never been alive, and therefore could not possibly be identical and have identical effects with those of the natural vitamin C one obtains from eating a tomato, a bell pepper or an orange.

Certainly the most cherished vitalistic concept—the one that all others appear to feed into—is that of postmortem survival, better known as "life after death." Even some of today's leading exponents of postmortem survival cast doubt on the validity of their beliefs. In the collection of "survivalist" essays entitled *What Survives?* (1990), Stanislav Grof, M.D., states that phenomena suggestive of postmortem survival "cannot be interpreted as unambiguous evidence for the continuity of individual consciousness after death." D. Scott Rogo writes that none of the cases cited in an essay he wrote "by itself proves that life extends beyond physical death," and that each case "suffers from certain evidential weaknesses or can be explained by theories other than psychic survival." Rupert Sheldrake, Ph.D., makes clear that his own survival-related hypothesis "does not automatically lead to the conclusion that . . . survival occurs." Ram Dass (Richard Alpert, Ph.D.) ascribes his "abundant" knowledge about alleged postmortem states of consciousness to his having heeded his "intuitive heart-mind . . . even though it is not open to the criteria of public reproducibility." Georg Feuerstein, M.Litt., admits: "Nothing can intellectually convince me that we survive physical death." Charles T. Tart, Ph.D., goes so far as to raise the question "Who Survives?" and suggests that persons who undertake "profound meditation and self-investigation" are the most likely to survive transition to an afterlife. In the same volume, Michael Grosso, Ph.D., suggests that resistance to vitalistic beliefs is motivated by such fears as "the primordial fear of hostile spirits," fear of hell ("moral and spiritual laziness"), and even "fear of enlightenment" (spiritual unpreparedness).

In spite of such self-criticism and flimsy rationalizing among believers, the scientifically obsolete vital-force hypothesis and its variants underlie a potpourri of fringe systems, modalities, and diagnostic methods. These include: "actualism," alchemical medicine, the Alexander technique, amulet healing, Anthroposophical medicine, applied kinesiology (including "muscle-testing"), behavioral kinesiology, aromatherapy, Aston patterning, attitudinal healing, aurasomatherapy, auriculotherapy, autogenics (autogenic training and autogenic therapy), Ayurvedic medicine and yoga, BioSonics, theologian John Bradshaw's "soulful" psychology, the Edgar Cayce approach, chakra healing, traditional Chinese medicine (including acupuncture, tai chi, and medical Qigong), traditional (and often modern) chiropractic, Christian Science, clairvoyant diagnosis, color therapy (chromotherapy), the *Course in Miracles* movement, craniosacral therapy (also called cranial technique, cranial osteopathy, or craniopathy) and its chiropractic equivalent neural organization technique

(NOT), creative visualization, crystal gazing ("scrying"), crystal therapy, dianetics, dreamwork, Dr. Wayne Dyer's "awakened life" program, Arnold Ehret's "mucusless" diet healing system, the Ferreri technique (a combination of applied kinesiology and neural organization technique), firewalking, flower essence therapy, Gerson therapy, G-jo, kahuna healing (Hawaiian Huna and lomi-lomi) and other forms of shamanism, herbalism, holotropic therapy (holotropic breath therapy), homeopathy, iridology, jin shin, Kirlian diagnosis (aura analysis), the laying on of hands, live-cell analysis, macrobiotics, medical astrology (astrologic medicine), medical graphology, mesmerism, myotherapy (Bonnie Prudden technique), Natural Hygiene, naturopathy, nutripathy, past lives therapy, pathworking ("guided meditation"), Dr. M. Scott Peck's "psychology of evil," polarity balancing (polarity therapy), pranic healing, primal therapy and "rebirthing," psi healing, psionic medicine or psionics ("medical dowsing" plus homeopathic concepts), psychic dentistry, psychic surgery, psychometry, pyramid power, radiesthesia ("medical dowsing") and its gadgety counterpart radionics (also called psionics), reflexology (ear, hand, foot, and body), Reichian-based therapies (e.g., orgonomy and bioenergetics), Reiki, ritual healing, rolfing (structural integration or structural processing), sclerology, seiki-jutsu, shiatsu, theotherapy, therapeutic touch and noncontact therapeutic touch, Tibetan medicine, "toning" (a form of music therapy), Touch for Health (a combination of applied kinesiology and "acupressure touch"), transcendental meditation (TM) and Sidhi (advanced TM), transpersonal and Jungian psychology, urine therapy, the Vega method (electrodermal or bioelectric testing), Zarlen therapy, and zone therapy (a composite of acupressure, reflexology, and tool-massage).

Nutrition and dietetics figure importantly in many of these systems, and sometimes most peculiarly. For example, in the yoga-oriented *Spiritual Nutrition and The Rainbow Diet* (1986), Gabriel Cousens, M.D., states: "By putting foods of various colors over each chakra [spiritual center of the human body], I was able to determine which colors were most enhancing for each chakra." Cousens holds that, "differently colored foods act specifically to energize and balance their particular color-coded chakras" and thus can heal the organs and nerve centers associated with the chakras.

Freelance writer Scott Cunningham, author of *Magical Herbalism* (1982) and *The Magic in Food* (1990), advocates "The Magical Diet." In the latter book, he relates how a vegetarian under an "evil spell" was advised to eat meat, whereupon she consumed a hamburger at a fast-food restaurant. "The meat made her sick to her stomach," writes Cunningham, "but it also ended the 'psychic attack.'" Cunningham recommends eating fresh mangos to stimulate sexual desire, and ripe mulberries to gain wisdom or to help increase "psychic awareness." In his *Chinese System of Food Cure: Prevention and Remedies* (1986), Henry C. Lu, Ph.D., recommends eating fifteen to twenty-five oysters with meals to cure tuberculosis of the lymph nodes and goiter—or one may use oyster sauce as seasoning if fresh oyster is not on hand. In *Crystal Power: The Ultimate Placebo Effect* (1989), critic Lawrence E. Jerome cites the claim that crystals, if used with herbs and a "properly prescribed" diet, can replace insulin injections for diabetics. Jerome adds that he knows of two people who died as a result of this substitution. *Jean Simpson's Numbers Diet* (1990) is described on the book's cover as a nutritionally sound, "diet-by-the-numbers" way to lose weight, based on the same idea behind the author's previous books, *Hot Numbers* and *Hot Lotto Numbers*. This approach is numerology, a vitalistic pseudoscience associated with witchcraft. Simpson claims that by using numbers based on the dieter's last birthday, she "can predict the kinds of diet downfalls that are most likely to occur on each Diet Day." *The Aquarian Guide to the New Age* (1990) states that "numerology is not always taken seriously, even among occultists." But "New Age" believers discriminate little.

What is Holism?

Most of the above-mentioned fringe systems and methods operate under the banner of "holism." "Holistic" or "alternative" medicine encompasses: (1) natural, Green, or Earth medicine; (2) folk, traditional, or planet medicine; (3) vibrational or energy medicine; and (4) occult medicine. Occult medicine includes: (1) direct, metaphysical, psychic, or spiritual "healing" and (2) "self-actuated healing," or "self-healing." *Holistic Health Promotion: A Guide for Practice* (1989) defines holism as "the view that an integrated whole has a reality independent of and greater than the sum of its parts." In the preface, the authors describe the neologism *bodymind* as "the most accurate expression of body-mind-spirit responses and experiences of being human." They define "healer" as:

> One who facilitates another person's growth toward wholeness (body-mind-spirit) or who assists with recovery from illness or transition to peaceful death. *Healing* is the process of bringing parts of oneself (physical, mental, emotions, spirit, relationships, and choices) together at deep levels of inner knowing, leading to integration and balance, with each part having equal importance

and value. This process is also referred to as self-healing or wholeness.

In the "New Age classic," *The Aquarian Conspiracy* (1980), Marilyn Ferguson writes: "The search for self becomes a search for health, for wholeness—the cache of sanity and wisdom that once seemed beyond our conscious reach. If we respond to the message of pain or disease, the demand for adaptation, we can break through to a new level of wellness." She later states that illness "is potentially transformative because it can cause a sudden shift in values, an awakening." But, according to the author, "every metaphor is potentially a literal reality" and the brain "has a kind of dark genius, organizing disorders appropriate to our most neurotic imaginings." Ferguson seems to be saying that disease is the body's way of telling us to straighten out.

"Holism" is a misnomer for what underlies unscientific medicine. Briefly, holists claim that "orthodox" medicine is preoccupied with the body and ignores the mind. Holists thus take for granted that mind and body interact somehow as independent entities—that they are two different things, rather than two aspects of a single phenomenon. Put another way, they assume that mental phenomena are not entirely dependent upon physiological processes. Besides being mistaken, this is actually a dualistic premise, diametric to holism. (It is properly called interactionism.)

Many proponents of "alternative" medicine say that the "interaction" of body and mind—or of body, mind, and spirit—should be the foremost concern of health professionals. In the September 1989 issue of *Edges*, a Canadian "New Age" quarterly, internist Richard Gerber, M.D., author of *Vibrational Medicine*, characterizes human beings as "multidimensional spiritual beings of light." "Vibrational healing modalities," he explains, "deliver specified quanta of subtle energy to promote healing through reintegration and realignment of our mind/body/spirit complexes. [They] work by rebalancing disturbances of structure and energy flow within the context of our multilevel interactive energy fields."

In an increasingly materialistic world, truly holistic "healing" systems are rare. They appear to foster solipsism, which is the view that all reality is a figment of the only thing that "really" exists—one's consciousness. Christian Science, a full-fledged religion, may be considered holistic because it maintains that the human body is not a physical entity at all and hence cannot fall ill. Its founder, Mary Baker Eddy (1821-1910), was apparently addicted to morphine and wholly rejected the scientific method. A declining carryover from the last "New Age," Christian Science has been called the oldest "mind-is-all" religion. It holds that reliance on medicine is sinful, and it disdains nearly anything that smacks of medicine. Unlike the world's major religions, Christian Science is utterly unconcerned with diet and nutrition. Eddy's scripture, *Science and Health* (1875), is used with the Bible to teach that pain and death are illusory. Christian Science has a worldwide membership, but in recent years has been beset by state prosecutors and internal dissent.

Christian Science "practitioners" are allegedly able to bring about resurrections. Yet a study published in the *Journal of the American Medical Association* in 1989 came to the conclusion that graduates of Principia College in Illinois—a four-year liberal-arts school for observant Christian Scientists—have a significantly higher mortality than graduates of a nonsectarian Midwestern college, even though Christian Scientists are forbidden to use tobacco or alcoholic beverages. Another study, published in 1991, compared the mortality of Principia alumni with that of Loma Linda University alumni. Most students at Loma Linda are Seventh-day Adventists, for whom use of tobacco and alcoholic beverages is likewise proscribed. However, Seventh-day Adventists also tend to consume little or no meat. This time, the Principia alumni fared even worse in the mortality-rate comparison.

Following Christian Science, *A Course in Miracles*, the voluminous bestseller supposedly channeled by "Jesus" through psychologist Helen Schucman (1909-1981), spawned a movement within a movement. The *Course*'s philosophy is holistic in that it upholds the Hindu notion that time and the physical world are illusions. Unlike Christian Science, the "Course in Miracles" movement is right at home in the sphere of "alternative" medicine.

In *The Greening of Medicine* (1990), Dr. Patrick C. Pietroni, past chairperson of the British Holistic Medical Association, acknowledges that some "alternative" medicine activities falter "on the edge of deceit and charlatanism" and that the term "holistic" has been "taken over by the alternative movement to the extent that it has lost . . . its original meaning."

The Placebo Effect

Psychosomatic ("mind-body") medicine is a legitimate branch of scientific health care. It is concerned mainly with physical disorders caused or aggravated by emotional disturbances. Prolonged stress, whether internal or external in origin, can result in a physical disturbance such as a peptic ulcer, high blood pressure, asthma, and dermatitis. Many "alternative" modalities share this focus, either openly or silently, with psychosomatic medicine. But proponents of "alternative" medicine trivialize, obfuscate, fail to acknowledge—or vastly overvalue—the commonest psychosomatic mechanism in their field: the placebo effect. If an improvement in health occurs after treatment (and if there is a causal relationship between these events), the improvement may be due largely to the patient's belief in the practitioner and/or therapy, rather than to the intrinsic worth of the therapy. This is called the "placebo effect," wherein "placebo" refers to any activity or substance that is either ineffective or nonspecifically effective relative to a given condition of a living organism. The abatement of such symptoms as poor appetite, constipation, dizziness, headache, backache, indigestion, insomnia, and tiredness, may be trumpeted as evidence that the patient has been "cured"—even while a life-threatening disease worsens. In *Follies and Fallacies in Medicine* (1990), Drs. Petr Skrabanek and James McCormick write:

> In the end it matters little whether a healer believes that he acts as a channel for the power of God or that he is an unrecognized Galileo who has discovered "natural" healing energy or that he sets out to gull the gullible: the means employed are of the same kind. The variety and absurdity of "alternative" cures is a tribute to the power, largely unrecognized and unacknowledged, of the placebo effect.

In the September/October 1992 *East West Natural Health*, Andrew Weil, M.D., author of *Natural Health, Natural Medicine* (1990), writes that he is "a great fan of placebo responses, considering them to be the heart of medical practice. It is in the interests of both doctors and patients to foster this kind of natural healing as often as possible."

Karl Sabbagh writes: "Any scientific explanation of the occasional effectiveness of fringe medicine is more likely to lie in the realms of orthodox psychology and physiology than in the more exciting worlds of forces, energy fields, meridians, and vibrations."

You, the Guinea Pig

An interwoven feature of "alternative" medicine is its emphasis on empiricism. The word "empiricism" has several meanings. As part of scientific research, empiricism refers to observation—just one step in the scientific method. But in "holistic" circles it is frequently a euphemism for quackery, for holists tend to "unshackle" observation from the scientific method and uphold it as self-validating. "Unshackled," empiricism has been misused to "prove" vitalistic concepts. For example, leading macrobiotics exponent Michio Kushi purports to demonstrate the existence of "chakras" by using nail clippers dangling from a thread (see Chapter 3). The unscientific empiricist will say that if the clippers move in a particular way, chakras exist.

The word "science" derives from the Latin verb *scire*, "to know." A scientist may be defined as an expert who pursues knowledge by means of the "scientific method." Scientists make tentative observations; collect data; construct testable hypotheses based on the data; test the hypotheses under stringently controlled, repeatable conditions; observe results; record results unambiguously; interpret them intelligibly; and actively seek criticism from other scientists and experts.

Scientists are also defined by what they eschew, including: (1) retention or reinstatement of a disproved theory for moral or pragmatic reasons; (2) "playing another ball game" by rejecting the accepted principles and procedures of the scientific method; (3) invocation of myths as evidence; (4) selection and organization of data to support a particular bias; (5) formulation of untestable hypotheses; (6) assignment of equal weight to all published reports, regardless of their quality or compatibility with the overall body of scientific knowledge; and (7) dogmatism. Christian Science, creation science, mytho-science, Vedic science, yoga science, and any "science" designated divine, esoteric, occult, sacred, or spiritual, are all oxymorons.

The above-mentioned pitfalls roughly reflect the "marks of pseudoscience" put forth by Daisie Radner and Michael Radner in *Science and Unreason* (1982). These pitfalls hindered Western medicine until about the turn of the century. Traditional Indian and Chinese systems of medicine did not fare nearly so well: they stagnated centuries ago and remain mixtures of science, religion, and fanciful physiology.

Scientists use empiricism, meaning observation, as *part* of the scientific method. Nonscientists regard it as experience and as adequate in itself. In medical practice, unscientific empiricists use experience as a substitute for scientific knowledge in selecting or improvising therapies. Empiricists reject scientific testing of their opinions and believe that their own clinical observations are more valuable than stringently controlled, peer-reviewed experiments. In *Health and Healing: Understanding Conventional and Alternative Medicine* (1983), Andrew Weil, M.D., writes: "The practical urgencies of illness do not permit the luxury of scientific contemplation. They demand immediate action." This view is fallacious.

Years ago, some surgeons thought they had developed a cure for angina pectoris, a type of chest pain associated with an insufficient supply of blood to the heart. Tying off an artery inside the chest apparently provided relief. But application of the procedure was short-lived, as subsequent research showed that a sham operation consisting of just a superficial incision on the chest wall was equally beneficial.

Even without paranormal underpinnings, empiricism can lead self-styled "scientists" to conclusions far afield of those based on extensive scientific experimental data. For example, in *Dismantling a Myth: The Role of Fat and Carbohydrates in Our Diet* (1987), internist Wolfgang Lutz claims that it is prudent to limit carbohydrate consumption to 80 grams per day. Lutz writes: "The best way of convincing a layman of the correctness of an idea is by an experiment involving his own person." In the chapter titled "Myself as the Guinea-Pig," he adds:

> As it should be, I began my experiments on myself. Although it is frowned upon in scientific circles to place too much weight upon personal observations, it is equally obvious that the most convincing evidence for a doubting scientist is what he can observe on himself. Even the most thorough and objective report of observations on others are no substitute for this.
>
> What I observed on my own person was so exciting that it is not easy to find words in which to describe this experience.

Lutz sympathizes with Robert C. Atkins, M.D., who, like Lutz, has promoted a high-fat/saturated fat, high-cholesterol, high-protein, very low-carbohydrate diet. Such a diet is likely to cause fatigue and uricemia, and increases the risk of heart disease and cancer. Regarding Atkins, see Chapter 7.

Matters of Faith?

Why do relatively few scientists and health professionals systematically examine "alternative" modalities based on empiricism and/or vitalistic concepts? Why is there no outcry from the scientific community and the health professions? It seems that, for most people, critical investigations of supernaturalistic claims are unrewarding both personally and financially. In *Crystal Power: The Ultimate Placebo Effect*, Lawrence E. Jerome writes:

> As a scientist, I've had to be a skeptic—to doubt, to question, to put to the test, to see evidence and proof. As a seeker of esoteric

knowledge, I've found myself hoping for the experiments to come out in favor of the crystals. . . .

After all, if I could find scientific evidence that crystal power actually exists, this book would find a ready and enthusiastic audience among the thousands, if not millions, of New Age practitioners, followers, and believers.

The World Almanac Book of the Strange (1977) suggests another reason for the reticence of scientists and health professionals:

This prejudiced attitude is not a conspiracy—as paranoid occultists are too likely to assume. The attitude stems, rather, from an understandable desire not to waste time and reputation in an area filled with crooks, cranks, and paranoid occultists. One scientist who made thorough tests of pyramid power and spoke of his negative findings to a group of believers was told, "You must have done something wrong or your pyramids would have worked." A scientist can have only one or two experiences like that before he decides that these are matters of faith, not science, and best left to believers.

Religion is a universal phenomenon both historically and geographically, and the desire to believe in the supernatural can be very strong. In *Wings of Illusion* (1990), clinical psychologist John F. Schumaker writes that no human trait is as widespread and pervasive as belief in the supernatural. He proposes that supernaturalistic beliefs have been "of such great survival value that, through evolution, we became biologically *predisposed* to believe the unbelievable." Schumaker calls this predisposition the "paranormal belief imperative"; philosophy professor Dr. Paul Kurtz calls it the "transcendental temptation."

"Alternative" medicine is a quasi-secular repository of supernaturalism. Supernaturalism holds that there are powers outside the universe or natural world, which at least occasionally affect courses of events. Vitalistic, theistic, and other supernaturalistic assumptions infuse "alternative" medicine, which, as a rule, represents disease as ultimately spiritual in nature, and which refers to occult and psychic concepts that defy scientific examination and measurement. Specifically, "alternative" medicine is characterized by: (1) dependence on alleged "psychic anatomies" such as the Hindu chakra system, the Chinese system of acupuncture meridians, and the supposed "astral body," "etheric body," or human "aura"; (2) the use of unscientific gadgets; (3) a desire to redefine science into conformation with a spiritist perspective; and (4) a refusal to rethink or repudiate a "treatment" in the face of scientific disproof. In contrast, naturalism is the basis of science and scientific medicine. It holds that the universe or natural world is all there is, and that all phenomena are explainable, at least in principle, without recourse to supernaturalistic concepts.

I believe that any "healing" system or modality that refers to alleged supernatural phenomena or makes common sense its primary recourse is seriously flawed. Supernaturalistic health-care philosophies may be entertaining and uplifting, and a commonsense approach to self-care comforting, but both are poor substitutes for medical science sagely applied. In any case, fringe health care is often oppressive and unsettling, and does not necessarily contribute to even a *sense* of well-being. Yet its appeal seems to lie in its ability to instill hope, allay fears, and generate purposefulness. Thus, I think of supernaturalistic and empirical health-care philosophies as religions. Alas, like many well-defined religions, they may also cause hardship, induce guilt, and foster elitism.

The Bottom Line

About fifty years ago, philosopher-scientist Bertrand Russell advised "giving to every suggested belief the degree of credence that the evidence warrants." But some Americans love hogwash so intractably that even (or especially) when their lives hang in the balance, they seem quite unable to distinguish hogwash from firm footing. I submit that "alternative" medicine is a no man's land of dangers—some obvious, others reasonably suspected, and yet others dimly conceived.

Our tour of the nutritional twilight zone, a region more of shadow than of substance, begins in the following chapter with a visit to the macrobiotic Kushi Institute.

3

Macrobiotics: "Livin' Large" ... or Largely Living?

Destination: Mecca

Macrobiotics, a comprehensive metaphysical system focused on diet and health and emphasizing self-care, was the apple of my eye in 1988. My appreciation of it was heightened, but also made skeptical, by Ronald Kotzsch's *Macrobiotics: Yesterday and Today* (1985), an insightful but partisan history of the movement. Kotzsch holds a doctorate from Harvard in the history of religions. The book is an outgrowth of his dissertation, "George Ohsawa and the Japanese Religious Tradition." In it I learned of the Vatican-like epicenter of macrobiotics—the Kushi Institute.

"Sounds Like Hocus-Pocus"

During the 1980s, the Kushi Institute had two locations in Massachusetts: a headquarters in Brookline (part of Boston) and the Kushi Institute of the Berkshires—once called Mt. Kushi Seminary. Recently, the Brookline facility was closed. Proponents anticipate that the Berkshire center, located on six hundred acres in Becket, will expand into a "One Peaceful World Village."

In June 1989, I attended the five-day Michio Kushi Seminar for Medical Professionals, held in Becket. A tall, thin, youthful macrobiotic convert and former marathon runner in his late forties met me at the bus station with a car. (I will refer to him below as "John," although that is not

23

his real name.) He was "interning" at the institute and had been following a macrobiotic diet for six months. As we awaited two other registrants, John described how the events following a diagnosis of cancer seven months earlier had led him to macrobiotics:

> Going and laying on that stainless steel table and getting these little lines drawn on me, I felt like a piece of beef. I felt like I had no control when they were getting ready to do radiation and the chemo. I went to see the oncologist, and seeing the other people in the waiting room, [I wondered], "Man, is that what I'm going to be looking like?" I mean, they didn't look well. They did not look healthy. . . . If I had done chemo and radiation, I know for a fact I wouldn't be sitting here having energy with you right now.

Ten days after receiving what he called the "verdict" of cancer from his primary physician, an endocrinologist, John had accepted two books from friends: *Recalled By Life* (1982), by Anthony J. Sattilaro, M.D., and *Confessions of A Kamikaze Cowboy* (1987), by actor Dirk Benedict. Both authors said they had recovered from cancer while following a macrobiotic regimen. Dr. Sattilaro (1931-1989), whose struggle with prostate cancer was widely publicized, had undergone extensive conventional therapy but credited macrobiotics for his improvement. In *Living Well Naturally,* a 1984 sequel to his first book, he said that his doctors had pronounced him in a state of permanent remission. However, he died of his disease shortly after the seminar I attended.

John said he had felt good reading the books and had concluded that basically "food is everything." Two days after receiving them, he phoned the Kushi Institute and urgently requested an appointment with Michio Kushi. Within an hour and a half of making the call, he boarded a plane for Boston, seeking a cure and spiritual renewal. He said did not inform his endocrinologist of his decision to turn to macrobiotics, because the doctor had warned him against charlatans. In retrospect, John said, he felt the endocrinologist was a charlatan for taking his money without "fixing" him. His present primary physician was a homeopath.

I asked John whether Kushi had performed a physical examination. "Just looking at the face, looking at the arms . . . he can tell how far it's advanced," John replied. "Before my cancer was diagnosed, I remember looking at my hand, and this area right here was just blue and green as hell. It looked like a bruise."

"You're pretty clean; you're clean," John assured me, examining my hand. "But mine was really blue and greenish, and that is one of the signs of cancer. . . . This area right here [between the thumb and forefinger] is the small intestine. That was so damn sore—in most people it is . . . from bad eating—that I couldn't press it like that. But everything in the body corresponds. Right now, looking at my hands, which one is the redder of the two? Obviously. The tumor's on this side. It's discharging through an extremity."

John promised me that Kushi would furnish "material evidence" of the chakras [in Hindu philosophy, the centers of spiritual energy in the human body]: "He'll take a little thing, like a nail clipper, dangling [from a thread], and when he puts it over this area of the body where there is a chakra, that thing will start to rotate. For men, it goes clockwise; for ladies, it goes counterclockwise."

John made much of the concept of "discharge":

Michio [Kushi] says that chicken is one of the most difficult things to discharge. It'll stay in your cells for nine months. You eat a piece of chicken, you won't discharge it till nine months later. It's almost stronger than beef.

Part of my regimen was to do body scrubs, because a major organ of the body is the skin. And if you've got a lot of fat there, the toxins come to the surface, hit that fat, turn right around, and go right back into the bloodstream. So I was doing body scrubs with hot towels and really scrubbing hard. I was up here maybe three weeks, and my back just broke out, all discharged stuff coming out of the pores of the skin. . . .

The diet that I'm on is mucus-free, and I'm throwing off mucus like it's going out of style. That's discharge. That's just junk coming out of the system that's been there for years.

The other form of discharge is emotional, and for everybody it's a different experience. . . . I've had a lot of discharge through dreams. My dreams from the time I got here till the present have been chronologically regressive. . . .

The theory of macrobiotics is that the foods that you ate [in the past]—the memories are kind of locked or stored in [your] cells. And when you discharge those and bring them forward, you start to release those memories. And I found it to be true. It sounds like hocus-pocus, but all I can say is, try it.

I asked John whether Kushi had looked at his lab reports. He replied:

Sure. . . . You know, the last time I took my blood test in to him . . . one test was way the hell out of whack. But he said: "Don't worry about it. . . . You're still building the good blood and you're discharging the bad."

But it's early. It's premature in the diet. . . . I mean, this thing took a while to form; it's going to take a while to discharge it. You don't want to discharge it too fast, either, when you've got something bad. . . . That can be radical.

John also spoke of reincarnation:

Hell, no one's gonna live forever in this life. Michio said this life is very important, but the next one is also important. And I said, "Michio, what happens if somebody comes to you and you know by looking at them that they're not gonna make it, either by macrobiotics or by Western medicine?" He said, "I still tell them to do macrobiotics . . . whether they do it for twenty days [or] twenty years. . . . The main thing is, they've made that decision. [The enlightenment gained] makes it so much easier the next time [in the next incarnation]."

Macrobiotics was a lifetime proposition for John:

What happens sometimes—and there's where you've got to watch your arrogance—[is], after being on the macrobiotic diet, you can feel better than you've ever felt in your life. You'll feel like, "Hey, if I take a little bit of this [macrobiotically unhealthful food], it won't hurt me." And it won't. But if you do it over and over again, the cancer . . . is not necessarily cured. It might still be there, and you will hold it there for the rest of your natural life by eating macrobiotically. . . . But you start getting back on the bad stuff, and some of those cells might really start to run rampant.

George Ohsawa and the "Diet Seven Rice Cure"

George Ohsawa (also known as Yukikazu Sakurazawa) was born Nyoiti (or Nyoichi) Sakurazawa in Kyoto, Japan, in 1893, to a family of samurai class. He was the founder of present-day macrobiotics and author of three hundred books and booklets. His first book in English, *Zen Macrobiotics*, appeared in mimeographed form in 1960. He described it as "the key, in reality a guidebook, to the Kingdom of Heaven," and called his physiologic philosophy "the hygiene of Hygeia." (Hygeia was the ancient Greek goddess of health and has been associated with a lifestyle-oriented approach based on "natural laws.")

In *Zen Macrobiotics*, Ohsawa claimed that all disease could be completely cured in ten days. "You must be your own doctor," he advised, emphasizing the concept of personal responsibility for disease (*"mea culpa"*). He added that people who do not accept such responsibility "do not deserve" a complete cure and "must not" be cured.

The earliest version of the macrobiotic diet appeared in this book and became known as the Zen macrobiotic diet. Proponents claimed that adherence to it could overpower a wide range of illnesses they attributed to dietary excesses. The diet had ten progressively restrictive stages. The lowest stage consisted of 10 percent grains, 30 percent vegetables, 10 percent soup, 30 percent animal products, 15 percent fruits and salads, and 5 percent desserts. In each subsequent stage, the percentage of grains increased by ten, while percentages for other categories decreased. The fourth stage excluded fruit; the sixth stage, all animal products. In every stage, fluid intake was restricted to no more than eight ounces daily. The highest stage, "Diet No. 7," limited food intake to whole grains (especially brown rice, the "principal food") and as little liquid as possible—in the form of mineral water, cereal beverage, or herbal tea. Ohsawa described Diet No. 7 as "the easiest, simplest, and wisest" way to well-being. Kotzsch notes that "the diet promised a quick fix—perfect physical and mental health, plus some species of enlightenment—in the ten days of the Diet Seven rice cure."

Ohsawa ardently supported French "scientist" Louis C. Kervran's unproven theory of biological transmutation of the elements. Kervran's *Biological Transmutations* was first published in 1962 and appeared a decade later in an English translation by Michel Abehsera, an Ohsawa disciple. Kervran held, for example, that silicon and carbon could combine in the presence of a specific enzyme to produce calcium. Indeed, he claimed that dietary calcium is virtually useless to the organism, especially in hot weather, and recommended ingestion of potassium and particularly "organic silica" (as in the diuretic herb horsetail) to strengthen bones. Believing in such alchemy to the extent of co-authoring a book on the subject with Kervran, Ohsawa was evidently quite unconcerned with adequacy of intake of specific nutrients.

From Ronald Kotzsch's panoramic history of the movement, Ohsawa emerges as a Japanese Don Quixote, preaching the "Unique Principle" of yin and yang and admonishing all to "chew very well." According to Kotzsch, Ohsawa identified the aim of macrobiotics as the achievement of "the health and freedom to be able to eat exactly what one wants." It seems that Ohsawa achieved this objective. Kotzsch writes that he occasionally enjoyed cheesecake, doughnuts, Coca-Cola, coffee, Guinness Stout, and Scotch whiskey, and was a heavy smoker "who for forty years taught about health with a cigarette in his hand." In *Macrobiotics: The Way of Healing*, Ohsawa claimed that tobacco smoking could both prevent and cure cancer.

Ohsawa spent about a year in India and became convinced that Ayurvedic medicine corresponded to macrobiotic practice. In 1955, he journeyed from India to what was then French Equatorial Africa to endeavor to convert Nobel laureate Dr. Albert Schweitzer to macrobiotics. During his stay at Schweitzer's mission, Ohsawa went about barefoot like the natives—and thus contracted filariasis, a tropical disease caused by a parasitic worm. Regarding drugs as "the devil's bullets," he refused medical intervention. In *Zen Macrobiotics,* Ohsawa declared that he had overcome his disease in a few days through macrobiotics. However, at age 72, he died of a heart attack that his doctor attributed to filarial infestation.

Why did Ohsawa shun medical treatment? In *Macrobiotics: The Way of Healing,* he professed: "Avoiding the consequences of . . . disease through artificial means would be cowardly. . . . One must see the disease through and overcome it without killing. The germs . . . must be allowed to live peacefully. Killing to defend oneself is not just."

The Aquarian Guide to the New Age (1990), a dictionary of pop metaphysics, states that macrobiotics "enjoyed a considerable fad in the West (where the system is still followed by a minority of alternative thinkers) but declined in popularity following the death from starvation of certain wealthy Americans who misunderstood its principles and failed to balance their food intake effectively." Kotzsch's book describes how, in 1965, a young woman in New York who had followed Diet No. 7 died "from an apparent combination of malnutrition and dehydration." As a result of her death, Ohsawa was sued and the Ohsawa Foundation in New York City was closed after an FDA raid. In 1967, the *Journal of the American Medical Association (JAMA)* presented a detailed account of a case of scurvy and malnutrition induced by fanatical adherence to a restrictive macrobiotic regimen. This article set the tone for orthodox medicine's view of macrobiotics. In 1971, the American Medical Association Council on Foods and Nutrition said that followers of the diet, particularly the highest stage, stood in "great danger" of malnutrition [*JAMA* 218:397, 1971].

The Kushi Era

Ohsawa's successor, Michio Kushi, was born in Japan in 1926. He met George Ohsawa in 1948 while studying international law at the University of Tokyo. He became Ohsawa's disciple, and first came to the United States in 1949 to attend graduate school at Columbia University. According to Kotzsch, Kushi read the manuscript for *Zen Macrobiotics*, expressed misgivings to Ohsawa regarding the strictness of the diet, and recommended changes—without success. During the 1960s Kushi settled in the Boston area and founded Erewhon, a distributor of "natural" and macrobiotic foods. In 1971, he established *East West Journal*, a monthly magazine; in 1972, the East West Foundation; and in 1978, the Kushi Institute. In 1982, the Kushi Foundation was established as the parent organization for the Kushi Institute and the magazine (renamed *East West Natural Health* in 1992).

Kushi is widely considered the foremost authority on macrobiotics. In *AIDS, Macrobiotics, and Natural Immunity* (1990), he recommends limiting consumption of: (1) fresh white-meat fish ("if needed or desired") to 1 to 3 days per week (5 to 10 percent of the day's food consumption); (2) fruit or "fruit desserts" to two or three servings per week; and (3) lightly roasted nuts and seeds to "occasional" status. He advises against frequent intake of any fruit juice, and recommends excluding virtually all foods of animal origin, most beverages other than water and certain herbal teas, virtually all processed foods, and hot spices.

In addition to holding lectures, seminars, and conferences, the Kushi Institute markets over a hundred books, audiotapes, and videotapes about macrobiotics and other topics consistent with its teachings. It also offers a Leadership Studies Program. Institute publications state that more than a thousand people around the world have attended classes at Brookline and Becket and graduated from this program. Similar programs have been offered by affiliated institutes in Amsterdam, Antwerp, Florence, Lisbon, London, and Kiental (Switzerland). Additionally, there are said to be six hundred macrobiotic "centers" located worldwide, one of which is the Macrobiotic Center of New York.

East West Natural Health has a circulation of about 100,000 and contains about 150 pages per issue. Its news and feature articles cover health, nutrition, psychology, and environmental issues—all from the macrobiotic perspective. Its editorial philosophy is antagonistic toward scientific medicine and certain public health measures, including fluoridation. Nonscientific systems such as acupuncture, chiropractic, Christian Science, homeopathy, naturopathy, and past-life therapy are promoted in uncritical articles. Full-page ads appear frequently for food supplements, herbs, "natural" cosmetics, and subliminal tapes. Classified ads involve such offerings as astrology and numerology reports; "consciousness in a bottle"; psychic readings; magnet therapy supplies; "mind expansion" videos; and correspondence courses in "divine science," "holistic healthcare," herbal medicine, hypnotherapy, iridology, nutrition counseling, and radionics.

Less of a "grand planner" than Kushi, America's second major macrobiotic guru— "Arm Chair Quarterback for the West," according to a 1989 ad—is Herman Aihara. Aihara was not only another of Ohsawa's early disciples, but Kushi's business partner and a pioneer marketer of rice cakes in the United States. His Japanese-born wife, Cornelia (also known as Chico Yokota), is also a macrobiotics teacher.

In *Acid and Alkaline* (1980), Herman Aihara asserts that, "theoretically," we are immortal, and cites the controversial experiment of Alexis Carrel, in which chick embryo cells apparently were kept alive for thirty-four years (see Chapter 11). In the early 1970s, Aihara established the George Ohsawa Macrobiotic Foundation (GOMF) to replace New York's Ohsawa Foundation. GOMF operates the Vega Study Center; sells macrobiotic foods, books, and other supplies; and publishes the bimonthly *Macrobiotics Today* and the works of Ohsawa and the Aiharas. GOMF and the center are located together in Oroville, California. The Vega Study Center was founded in the mid-1980s and holds macrobiotic conferences, counselor training forums, Shinto ceremonies, and potluck lunches. *Macrobiotics Today* has a circulation of about three thousand.

Scores of books and numerous articles have been published lauding macrobiotics. *Macrobiotic Miracle: How a Vermont Family Overcame Cancer* (1984), for example, is a testimonial co-authored by Virginia Brown, formerly a registered nurse for thirty-five years. Brown says that familiarity with the Edgar Cayce tradition paved the way for her acceptance of macrobiotics. And in *The Way of Life: Macrobiotics and the Spirit of Christianity* (1986), Episcopal priest John Ineson seeks to reconcile Christianity with macrobiotics.

What Is Macrobiotics?

Kotzsch says it is unclear how the term "macrobiotics" occurred to Ohsawa, but speculates that it may have come from the title of a book by an eighteenth-century German physician, Christoph Wilhelm von Hufeland. Von Hufeland posited that proper cultivation of the "Life Force"—which he claimed was absorbable from food—was the key to health and longevity. The measures he espoused are very similar to those propounded by Natural Hygiene (covered in Chapter 4). In *Are You Confused?*, originally published in 1971, naturopath Paavo Airola (1915-1987) wrote: "Ohsawa merely borrowed the word originated by Hufeland and built his own dietary system around it, giving it an oriental touch."

The French version of *Zen Macrobiotics* was published in 1961 as *Zen Macrobiotique*—literally, "macrobiotic Zen." In both the French and English versions of the book, the emphasis was on the word "Zen." *You Are All Sanpaku*, a so-called version for the general public, was published in 1965. Its author was William Dufty, who later wrote *Sugar Blues* (1975), a diatribe against the consumption of sugar. In an interview in the Summer 1989 issue of *Solstice*, an independent (now defunct) macrobiotic magazine, Dufty stated:

> The mystery is, how did this French adjective get to be a plural noun in English? . . . How it came to mean an open-ended abstract noun with horrible resonances, which provokes an impression at polar length from that which it means to convey . . . [is] beyond me. The people around George Ohsawa had not a sufficient command of their own language, let alone a second one. If macrobiotics had chewed these words instead of brown rice, the miasma of confusion from using the word as a plural abstract would never have existed. . . . Using the word as a noun is garbage. . . . I don't want to have anything to do with the word.

The word "macrobiotic" is derived from the Greek *macrobiotos*—"long-lived." Macrobiotics literally means "large" or "long" (*macro*) life (*biotics*). Descriptive definitions abound, yet a satisfactory "nuts and bolts" definition of the concept does not come easily. A definition in *The New Age Dictionary* (1990), edited by Alex Jack, a macrobiotics teacher and former editor-in-chief of *East West*, is ascribed to Michio Kushi:

> The way of health, happiness, and peace through biological and spiritual evolution and the universal means to practice and harmonize with the Order of the Universe in daily life, including the selection, preparation, and manner of cooking and eating, as well as the orientation of consciousness toward infinite spiritual realization.

A definition five paragraphs long, but described as short, appeared in the December/January 1989 *Solstice*. It states that macrobiotics is "a way of living with respect for the physical, biological, emotional, mental, ecological, and spiritual order of our daily lives . . . . not a particular form of therapy or medicine. . . . not a religion." In contrast, a 1974 *Nutrition Today* article described macrobiotics as a cult and as a "religion with strong dietary overtones"—a fitting impression, since its underpinnings include Zen Buddhism, Hinduism, and Shinto, the aboriginal religion of Japan.

These underpinnings are criticized by Kotzsch, who cites "an assumed identity between 'macrobiotic' and 'traditional Japanese' culture." In an interview in the March/April 1989 *Solstice*, he acknowledged the religious nature of macrobiotics and cited the need for a "nonideological" version. Kotzsch further acknowledges:

> There is no explicit, generally accepted understanding of what it means to be "macrobiotic." Macrobiotics is many-faceted. It includes a diet, a system of medicine, a philosophy, a way of life, a community, and a broad social movement.

Ohsawa offered a simple, if obscure, definition in *Macrobiotics: An Invitation to Health and Happiness* (1971): "To live in perpetual ecstatic delight is Do-o-Raku. Those who do so are called Do-o-Raku-Mono. If you are Do-o-Raku-Mono, you are Macrobiotic, whatever you eat."

In the *Solstice* interview, Kotzsch suggested that a shift in emphasis toward healing started in the early 1970s: "I remember Michio saying that if macrobiotics demonstrated that it could cure cancer, it would attract attention and influence many people." Kushi has predicted that the modern scientific orientation will be discarded within fifty to seventy years and replaced by "a new science, based on a dynamic understanding of natural order and the unifying principle of yin and yang." In *The Macrobiotic Approach to Cancer* (1991), Kushi states that cancer and other diseases are caused mainly by imbalances of "yin" and "yang" produced by a faulty diet.

Yin and Yang Upside-Down

According to ancient Chinese cosmology, yin and yang are the complementarily opposite cosmic principles or "energy modes" that compose the *Tao*. Usually translated as "The Way," the word *Tao* unifies three concepts: ultimate, all-embracing reality; universal energy; and living in harmony with the universe. The "heavens" are said to be yang and to represent the active, bright, male principle. The earth is yin and represents the passive, dark, female principle. But nothing is completely yin or yang. A given object or condition is yin or yang only relative to another object or condition. In *Acid and Alkaline*, Herman Aihara explains:

> Yin and yang are antagonistic but also complementary. Therefore, the yin-yang concept is not Western dualism which sees nature as two antagonisms: capitalist vs. labor, rich vs. poor, good vs. bad, right vs. wrong. . . . There is yin inside yang and there is yang inside yin.

Citing yin-yang theory, macrobiotics can relate itself to everything in the universe, encompassing every conception from world peace to sexual orientation. However, the relationship between macrobiotics and Chinese yin-yang theory is not clear-cut. Macrobiotics distinguishes according to structure, while the Chinese theory—which includes acupuncture theory—distinguishes by function. For example, macrobiotics classifies the earth (compact) as yang and the "heavens" (diffuse) as yin, while Chinese cosmology takes the opposite view. Furthermore, as noted by Dr. Louis E. Grivetti in the November/December 1991 issue of *Nutrition Today*, traditional Chinese medicine assigns neutrality to candy and categorizes salt as yin, whereas candy is yin and salt yang from the macrobiotic perspective. Traditional Chinese medicine also identifies certain domesticated animals—dogs, for instance—as especially nourishing foods. Thus, as Kotzsch notes, "while Ohsawa purports to present an ancient Oriental way of thinking, in practice his [system] does not correspond to the classical Chinese system."

In *Zen Macrobiotics*, Ohsawa gave cold and heat, expansion and contraction, outward and inward, up and down, purple and red, light and heavy, and water and fire as examples of yin and yang, respectively. He believed that whole grains, particularly brown rice, were near the midpoint of yin and yang. Macrobiotics classifies foods according to: (1) climate—hot yielding yin foods, cold yielding yang; (2) pH—acid is yin, alkaline yang; (3) taste—sweet vs. salty; (4) color—purple vs. red; and (5) water content—perishable vs. dry. But an orange, despite its yang color, is yin because it is cultivated in tropical and subtropical regions, and is acidic, sweet, and juicy. Orange juice is more yin because of its greater water content. Both foods are undesirable from a macrobiotic standpoint, especially for people living in colder regions, because they are too yin relative to whole grains.

In an article reprinted in the July/August 1991 *Macrobiotics Today*, Xander Steevensz, who was apparently "forced into" macrobiotics by his parents when he was about fourteen years old, describes his curious upbringing. Once, in response to his misbehavior, his parents made him copy by hand the entire contents of George Ohsawa's *Book of Judgment*. "Anything yin," he says, "was taboo—fruits were particularly forbidden—and meat was a cardinal sin." Thus, writes Steevensz, "junk food" became the "rebellious outlet" for himself and his sister. "You should never feel guilty when you consume foods too yin or too yang," Steevensz concludes. "All foods should enter your body with all your blessing and happy thoughts as well as good chewing. The point is, don't look for macrobiotic food, look for food macrobiotically"—that is, from the perspective of yin and yang. Steevensz's conclusion may leave one wondering whether "overdosing" on yang—say, wolfing down a cheese omelet—can be counteracted with a helping of an extremely yin dessert, such as pineapple frozen yogurt.

A substratum of yin-yang theory, Eastern religions, and Japanese culture complicates macrobiotics. But as far as diet is concerned, it boils down to the consumption of unprocessed or minimally processed foods, primarily whole grains and vegetables, which, ideally, should be grown "organically" in the region where the consumer lives and eaten in season. *Health Foods Business* estimates that total 1988 sales of macrobiotic foods through "health food" stores were $29.8 million.

The Seminar

Throughout the year, the Kushi Institute conducts residential seminars ranging from weekend workshops to its five-week Leadership Studies Program. The seminar I attended cost $450, which covered tuition, room, and board. However, upon registering, I was charged an additional $30 for membership in Kushi's nonprofit organization, One Peaceful World— required for participation in all institute programs. While the accommodations were modest, the lush Berkshire Hills setting was breathtaking.

Eighteen people other than myself attended the seminar: twelve medical doctors, two registered nurses (one a nurse practitioner), an osteopath, an endodontist, a chiropractor, and a nutrition researcher with a doctorate. The M.D.s included a homeopath, an orthopedist, and a physician identified as a pioneer "clinical ecologist." The orthopedist complained that Western medicine was "so minutia-oriented." Two of the attendees were visibly overweight. One of the physicians said he had cancer. The attendees' experience with macrobiotics ranged from dabbling to ten years, but most attendees had been practicing macrobiotics for more than six months, and some had been practicing it for several years. They had come from as far as Michigan, Tennessee, and Ontario, Canada.

The Kushi Institute of the Berkshires had three main buildings: a rambling, multistory Main House, originally a hunting lodge and later a Christian monastery; a dormitory; and a house that includes a library, a kitchen, a dining room, and a temple. Orientation took place in the library after dinner. A tall, thin, self-possessed man named Charles Millman presided. He introduced our program host, Jimmy, who appeared to be in his late teens or early twenties. Jimmy had completed the third and highest level of the Leadership Studies Program after emigrating from Yugoslavia with his family. Then his parents, who ran the kitchen, were introduced. In broken English, Jimmy's father told us how his wife had recovered from ovarian cancer through macrobiotics. Three years earlier, he said, doctors had predicted that she would survive for only two to three months.

Next, Millman introduced the co-director of the center and plugged her recently published book-length testimonial. She said she had grown up with a deep appreciation for health professionals—because she had always been sick. But since 1982, she added, her only health problem had been a single headache. John was the last person introduced, and briefly told his story.

Each of us received a packet containing information on the diet, macrobiotic seminars and publications, traditional Chinese methods of diagnosis, the Kushis' nearby "natural food" store ("Aveline's," named after Michio's wife), and their macrobiotic Japanese restaurant (then called "Ghinga") in Stockbridge, Massachusetts. Millman informed us of Michio and Aveline's "grand plan" to turn the Berkshire facility into the world's macrobiotic educational nucleus—a One Peaceful World Center. He said: "By creating biological peace, by giving people health, you can create peace in various families, in various societies, nations, and throughout the world, spreading our teachings, and helping people to live healthy, happy lives." Later, he asked us to wash our own dishes and silverware. "This is not slave labor," he assured us, but "simply part of standard macrobiotic lifestyle practice, keeping everything very orderly and very neat."

In the dining room, the halves of the buffet were labeled "regular" and "medicinal." Foods on the latter half were purportedly lower in salt and intended for participants who had reported an illness prior to their arrival. The only visible sources of liquids were water faucets and two urns. One urn contained, as I recall, bancha tea (*kukicha*, or "twig tea"), and the other contained what was described as a coffee substitute, probably dandelion root tea. I was soon craving diet soda. The grain-centered diet provided during the seminar was bland-tasting and monotonous. Relative to the Recommended Dietary Allowances (RDAs), it appeared low in calcium, riboflavin, and vitamins B_{12} and D.

One evening I rushed through my brown rice and vegetables in anticipation of having my sweet tooth satisfied by a creamy-looking strawberry dessert, but it fell far short of my expectations. Most of the attendees, however, appeared to relish the food. One even remarked to a host: "If we have any more food like we've had in the last twenty-four hours, you'll have to roll us all down the hill." Fewer than forty-eight hours after my arrival, I could hardly wait to get home. I slept uncomfortably on a lumpy mattress, I was constipated (an unusual circumstance), and I had flu-like symptoms that disappeared only during my return trip to New York.

Bad Vibes, Condensed

The next morning, at 7:00, we commenced our daily exercise class in the library. Our instructor, Michael Joutras, said the exercises (called *Do-in*) affected the flow of energy (*ki* or *Ch'i*) through body channels (invisible "meridians"). These exercises, he said, share the system on which acupuncture and shiatsu (finger-pressure at acupuncture points) are based. He told us to rub our palms together. "Our hands are especially charged with energy," he said. "There's a meridian going through each finger. . . . Now hold your hands slightly apart. Can you feel any electrical sensation?" he asked. I couldn't. "If you can't, pull them slightly apart, then bring them in closer again." I still couldn't feel any electrical or other sensation. Finally, Joutras said: "If you can't feel it, that's okay."

He told us that while nutrition scientists focus mainly on the physical aspects of food—"vitamins, nutrients, fat, and so forth"—the Eastern view was broader:

So meat has a certain kind of energy. Sugar has a certain kind of energy. Dairy food has a certain kind of energy. And when we ingest these things, then that energy is going into our body, and being released through the process of digestion, and going through the whole body, carried through the meridian system. And so the underlying basis of sickness was always that energy is unbalanced.

Later he stated:

The definition of matter is . . . nothing but energy, and waves, and vibrations. . . . There is nothing but condensed vibration. . . . Everything is spirit. Everything is energy, condensed energy, different qualities of energy. Although we're all made up of organs and cells and blood vessels, everyone is still different, because everyone has a different energy, different vibration, or different soul or spirit or whatever you want to call it. . . . It's something that you really can't measure, although . . . intuitively we know it's there. But you really can't measure it, I don't think.

A "False Impression"?

Our daily cooking class began at 10:00 A.M. in the Main House. It was conducted by Wendy Esko, a thin, barefaced, forty-year-old woman with long hair, who said she had stumbled onto macrobiotics nineteen years previously and had been practicing it ever since. The class topic was "Medicinal Use of Food." Wendy cautioned us that vegetables prepared in a food processor could trigger hyperactivity in children.

Next came Martha Cottrell, M.D., a contributor to the pro-macrobiotic collection of essays, *Doctors Look at Macrobiotics* (1988)—edited by Wendy's husband, Edward Esko—and co-author with Esko and Michio Kushi of *AIDS, Macrobiotics, and Natural Immunity*. Cottrell called Kushi "psychic." "I've been macrobiotic pretty much for about ten years," she said. "I started when I turned fifty in 1978. Without any doubt, I feel that macrobiotics has given me at least ten years' additional life, and maybe more. And I want to use it well, and have fun doing it, too." Before turning to macrobiotics, she told us, she had suffered from arthritis, gastrointestinal problems, eczema, and psoriasis. But she noted that some macrobiotic leaders had not learned how to take care of themselves very well. "Michio is so driven by what he wants to do before he dies," she said. "I was in Florida with him not long ago, and he looked extremely tired. And he's still smoking."

After dinner, Millman plugged two macrobiotic cookbooks and Kushi's *Crime and Diet* (1987) before introducing Edward Esko, who looked anemic despite a mild facial sunburn. Esko lamented that macrobiotics was so misunderstood—"especially the whole Zen macrobiotic and brown rice diet," which he described as "actually twenty-five years out of date and . . . still on some people's minds." Then he told us that a writer (Stephen Harnish, M.D., a contributor to *Doctors Look at Macrobiotics*) had recently done a computerized literature search (using MEDLINE) and found twenty-three articles on macrobiotics. Twenty-one were negative. Esko declared that an equal number of positive articles needed to be published in medical journals to "counteract that false impression that many people have."

Esko said that Ohsawa had chosen the term "Zen" because of a rough connection with Buddhist vegetarian cooking, and because Zen philosophy had been popular at that time in New York. "So it was kind of a marketing strategy," he explained. Esko nonchalantly refuted Newton's Universal Law of Gravitation, stating that gravity simply doesn't exist. He expounded on the ancient Chinese theory of Five Elements and its relationship to macrobiotic yin-yang theory. According to ancient Chinese tradition, *Ch'i* or *Qi* ("life energy"), after arising from a primary energy source, differentiates into yin and yang. Yin and yang differentiate into the five "elements" (also called "phases" or "transformations") of which all things are made. These "elements" are earth, water, fire, wood, and metal.

Next, he introduced us to a young woman from Lima, Peru, who had long, beautiful hair. She said she had pursued macrobiotics after a magnetic resonance imaging (MRI) scan—a high-tech diagnostic procedure—had confirmed the presence of a brain tumor. She told us she had lost all her hair as a result of conventional cancer therapy. Refreshingly, at least two attendees inquired whether she had undergone another MRI scan (to verify her supposed cure) after adopting macrobiotics. She said she hadn't because her doctor had dispelled the option as an unnecessary expense.

"This Is No Gimmick"

Kushi did not appear until the third day of the seminar, at which time he lectured on diagnostic principles. His broken English often made him unintelligible.

"Modern medicine is physical, material way, analytical way," he said, "therefore overlooking this universe's force coming in, and the earth force go up, coming in constantly, constantly, constantly." To demonstrate this alleged force, Kushi produced nail clippers suspended from a dark thread. "This is no gimmick," he assured us. "It's a nail clipper. . . . This is just thread only." Then, dangling the clippers over a supine doctor, he proceeded to give the chakra demonstration John had promised during our conversation. Kushi said that the chakras caused the clippers to trace small circles over areas of the body corresponding to them. However, close observation revealed that the circling was caused by movements of Kushi's arm.

In yoga philosophy, the chakras are vortices that penetrate the human body and its "aura." They are supposedly the means by which the "universal life force" (*prana* or *Ch'i*) is transformed and distributed. Although there are alleged to be only seven major "body chakras," there is no consensus on the total number of chakras; hundreds of minor ones are believed to exist. In any case, there is no scientific evidence of their existence. But then, the methods espoused by Kushi do not correspond to scientific medical practice, but are part of what he calls the "traditional arts of Oriental healing." They include pulse diagnosis, visual diagnosis, meridian diagnosis, voice diagnosis, astrological diagnosis, parental and ancestral diagnosis, aura and vibrational diagnosis, consciousness and thought diagnosis, environmental diagnosis, and spiritual diagnosis—all of which were defined in the information packet we received.

Voice diagnosis supposedly identifies disorders of the glands, organs, and certain body systems. Kushi said, for example, that a "watery voice . . . means natural kidney-bladder is overworked. Also must be blood vessels expanded for too much water. . . . So when [you] hear a watery voice, then you should immediately know heartbeat overworked, and kidney overworked, and blood overworked."

Astrological diagnosis, as described in the information packet, uses the time and place of birth and current astrological and astronomical conditions to "characterize the basic constitutional tendencies of the body and the mind as well as the potential destiny of the current and future life of the subject." After outlining nine Oriental "astrological types," Kushi summoned volunteers representing "opposite" types, compared their smiles, and commented that some were "very idealistic, very romantic, uplifted" and fond of theatrics, while their supposed opposites were "gentle" and "more reserved." He remarked that members of each group had very similar smiles. "Face is very similar, right?" No one voiced disagreement, and Kushi went on unimpeded.

Behavior diagnosis supposedly reveals dietary imbalances impacting on behavior. For example, Kushi said that if one eats too much fish, the next day he will be making fish-like movements. He illustrated his point by sitting in a chair and moving his knees repeatedly apart and together. (Kushi's antic is analogous to the chicken "simmer sauce" commercial with the slogan "I feel like chicken tonight," in which people flap their arms like chicken wings in anticipation of dinner.)

Environmental diagnosis involves an examination of atmospheric conditions and celestial influences, supposedly to reveal the "environmental cause" of physical and psychological disorders. Kushi said that during sleep, one's head "should be more north if you are living in northern hemisphere. If you are living in southern, opposite."

After supper, before the lecture resumed, two doctors tried to duplicate Kushi's chakra demonstration. When I pointed out to one that her arm was moving, she invited me to try. I did, holding my arm still, and, as nothing happened, she responded: "Oh, my God, when somebody wants to, they can really botch this."

The next session opened not with Michio, but with his wife, Aveline, in traditional Japanese dress, discussing her recent translation of a Japanese fortuneteller's book on nutrition (published in 1991 as *Food Governs Your Destiny*). Following this, Millman proceeded to read the introduction to Aveline's work, and continued dutifully for eight-and-a-half minutes.

It was perhaps not by chance that the room was dim when Kushi performed a variation of the first chakra demonstration. The nail clippers dangled above the head of a female attendee seated on the floor with her eyes closed. He instructed her:

> Please just remain quiet, okay? . . . Please, very quiet, please. . . . Now, start to think again. . . . Think of husband or boyfriend. Or romance. Your partner. . . . Now, let's change content of thinking. Think about war. Many of friends is hurt. . . . Towns and cities are burned and destroyed. Many thousand, thousand people are being killed, and we are burning.

Kushi maintained that "by thought . . . the chakra vibration change[s]"—that the increasing speed of the circling reflected the increasing intensity of the woman's mental processes. As the nail clippers circled the alleged crown chakra, he asked questions about their motion, presumably distracting the audience from his arm movements.

When I last saw him, Kushi was exhorting the physicians to fulfill their true role as teachers of the macrobiotic way of life.

Macrobiotics and AIDS: "Death Is a Gateway"

In an interview in the May/June 1990 issue of *Spectrum* (formerly *Macrofax*), Kushi identified the cause of AIDS as excessive consumption of drugs, simple sugars, and foods high in fat. The ramifications of Kushi's views are revealed uncritically in Tom Monte's *The Way of Hope: Michio Kushi's Anti-AIDS Program* (1989). Monte, who also co-authored *Recalled By Life* with Dr. Anthony Sattilaro, describes macrobiotics as "a philosophical system grounded in diet," according to which "nothing happens in life that is arbitrary or unjust" and "death is a gateway." He portrays Kushi as a heroic missionary selflessly braving the medical establishment, organized religion, and, perhaps worst of all, a bleak gay subworld where "strange feelings" predominate and no one appears to know "how far is too far." He quotes a study participant who said that Kushi was perceived "as a messenger from God."

In *The Way of Hope*, Monte traces the origin and course of a small and far-from-conclusive study undertaken within the context of a macrobiotic support group for gay men with AIDS. He also describes the initiation of one such individual into macrobiotics by a former Kushi student who discouraged him from undergoing medical tests and chemotherapy as recommended by his physician. The gay man and his lover, also diagnosed with AIDS, went to Boston to consult Kushi. Kushi's final bit of advice to them was: "Every day, sing a happy song." No mention is made of the cost of the consultation. The first member of the support group to succumb had a tumor on his neck "the size of a grapefruit," which "had continued to grow." Another member refused painkillers despite "unbearable" pain.

The study began in May 1984 with ten gay male Manhattan residents diagnosed with AIDS and Kaposi's sarcoma. Its collaborators include Martha Cottrell and Kushi's son, Lawrence Haruo Kushi, who holds an M.S. degree from the Harvard School of Public Health. The study group enlarged, but the book does not make clear whether the maximum number of subjects was twenty or twenty-four. In any case, Monte quickly dismisses the fates of those other than the original ten. In a 1989 issue of *Brain, Behavior, and Immunity*, Cottrell and associates reported that the total number of subjects was nineteen and that as many as thirteen had died. According to the "natural health" magazine *Bestways*, only five of the original ten were still alive as of March 1990.

On September 17, 1992, I phoned one of the original study collaborators, Elinor M. Levy, Ph.D., at the Boston University School of Medicine. Levy stated that, at most, only two of the original ten subjects were still alive. One was doing well, and the other had been out of touch for a "few years." This result certainly does not support the idea that macrobiotic eating can help AIDS patients.

Incidentally, Monte avers that Kushi regards homosexuality as a question of choice and "has tended to be nonjudgmental in such matters." But, according to Kotzsch, Kushi "has maintained that homosexuality is a loss of natural balance and not just a matter of preference," and regards both male and female homosexuality as dietarily reversible "conditions." Kushi himself, in his *Book of Macrobiotics* (1984), classifies homosexuality as an "Endless Disorder."

Macrobiotic Self-Defeat

Lawrence Lindner, M.A., executive editor of the *Tufts University Diet & Nutrition Letter*, had a private consultation with Edward Esko at the Kushi Institute as part of an assignment for *American Health* magazine, and reported his findings in the May 1988 issue. Esko told him that: (1) excessive consumption of fruit had caused enlargement of his heart; (2) his kidneys were weak; (3) he was slightly hypoglycemic; (4) deposits of fat and mucus were starting to accumulate in his intestines; (5) cold drinks would freeze the deposits and produce kidney stones; and (6) he should avoid eating chicken because it is linked with pancreatic cancer and melanoma. The consultation cost $200. Lindner concluded, in part: "The macrobiotic lectures, courses, books and tapes . . . besides running into hundreds or thousands of dollars, teach a philosophy of life, not nutrient interactions." In an interview, he added: "Some people are attracted to macrobiotics because, like a typical cult, it seems to offer simple solutions to a variety of life's problems."

Studies have revealed significantly lower blood pressure readings and cholesterol levels among followers of macrobiotics. But without supplementation, a vegan diet—which excludes all foods derived from the animal kingdom—requires careful planning to ensure nutritional adequacy. While the macrobiotic diet is all-encompassing in theory, in practice it is nearly vegan, and tends to be low in iron, calcium, and vitamins B_{12} and D. Further, it is considerably more limited in food options than an ordinary vegan diet. It virtually excludes—just for example— citrus foods, bananas, honey, sugar, potatoes, tomatoes, and spinach. Over the years, many reports have noted iron and vitamin B_{12} deficiencies, rickets, retarded growth, and below-normal stature among children on the diet. Moreover, macrobiotic adults have been found to have low serum concentrations of B_{12}.

The riskiness of the diet increases for the ill, particularly persons with cancer or AIDS. Such persons have elevated energy and protein requirements, may get full quickly, and may experience increased fluid losses from diarrhea, vomiting, or sweating due to fever. In contrast, the macrobiotic diet tends to be low in calories, protein, and fluids, and its high fiber content is likely to exacerbate both early satiety and diarrhea. Several lawsuits have claimed that cancer patients who relied upon macrobiotics instead of proven therapy met with disaster.

Macrobiotic proponents respond to these criticisms in several ways. They say that nutritional deficiencies result only from following the diet incorrectly—in an overly restrictive fashion. They claim they do not try to lure patients away from medical treatment with promises that the diet will cure them. And they point to research findings suggesting that macrobiotics is protective against coronary heart disease. They are hardly likely to add, however, that other dietary approaches to disease prevention, such as the Pritikin diet or a well-balanced vegetarian diet, are nutritionally superior and likely to be much more palatable.

"Health food" advocate Annemarie Colbin, M.A., is founder and director of the Natural Gourmet Institute for Food and Health in New York City and a columnist for *Free Spirit*, a "holistic living magazine." In *Food and Healing* (1986), which she dedicated to George Ohsawa ("whose vision sparked mine"), Colbin offers this critique:

> Because macrobiotics as philosophy deals not only with proper eating, but also sets up general rules of conduct and judgments about the "true" conditions of health and the evils of the world, it often gives rise to arrogance in the teachers, fear and guilt in their followers—the very qualities that it pretends to abolish. It can thus defeat its own purpose.

Colbin concludes: "Food serves us best not as our master, but as our tool and instrument, our helper and facilitator."

The Bottom Line

No long-range study has been attempted to determine whether macrobiotic devotees wind up, on balance, better off than their nonmacrobiotic counterparts. Since macrobiotics represents a cauldron full of variables, such a study could be difficult to construct. To begin with, as Kotzsch has admitted, no one can state with precision what it means to be "macrobiotic." Moreover, if the results of such a study showed that devotees fared better, the reasons for their success might be extremely difficult to identify.

Although macrobiotic eating might improve the health of many American adults, it carries a significant and unnecessary risk of nutritional deficiencies. Nutrient supplementation, laboratory tests, and consultations with a qualified nutrition professional could minimize this risk. But macrobiotic philosophy discourages the use of such safeguards, and thus heightens the riskiness of the diet.

4

Hazardous "Hygiene"

"Health Care Is Self Care"

Natural Hygiene is a comprehensive philosophy of health and "natural living," central to which is a strict vegetarian (vegan) diet of uncooked vegetables, fruits, nuts, and seeds. According to Natural Hygiene, fasting is beneficial whether one is sick or healthy, and virtually all medical treatments are condemnable. The cover of a 1984 issue of *Vegetarian Health Science* identifies its fundamental teaching: "Health Care Is Self Care." Its allure for me, in 1989, lay in this teaching and in its emphasis on such simple preventive measures as consumption of fresh fruits and vegetables, moderate exercise, proper rest and sleep, and meaningful occupation.

Was Reverend Graham Crackers?

Proponent literature traces the emergence of "Hygiene" to the year 1820 and a God-fearing Connecticut physician named Isaac Jennings (1788-1874). Jennings taught that "obedience to physical law will render obedience to moral law comparatively easy." He was convinced that medicines were worthless and that providing the prerequisites for health was sufficient to prevent disease. According to the January/February 1992 issue of the Natural Hygienist magazine *Health Science*:

His loss of faith in drugs occurred while he was attending a young

45

woman afflicted with typhus fever. When it appeared that she might die, he discontinued the use of medication.

From a pure spring he obtained some water which he placed in a vial and gave to his patient in place of drugs. In a short time she began to improve, and shortly afterwards made a complete recovery.

In the same decade, an uneducated Silesian farmer, Vincenz Priessnitz (1799-1851), developed hydropathy ("water cure"), which later became confluent with "Hygiene." Today, hydro*therapy* is used in scientific medicine as a mode of physical therapy in which water is used externally in the treatment of speicific diseases. For example, a whirlpool bath may be used to soothe the aching joints of patients with arthritis. Priessnitz, however, promoted both internal and external use of water, particularly surface applications of ice-cold water, as something of a panacea. He believed that bacteria were more susceptible to cold than to heat, basing this belief on his observation that cold generally inhibited animal breeding. In 1826, he opened the Hydropathic Institution of Grafenberg, which became an international success despite its reportedly greasy food and squalid living quarters. Treatments included baths, the winding of wet sheets around the body, enemas, douches, and the dripping of water on ailing parts of the body. The most formidable component of Priessnitz's regimen was the "douche bag"—a stream-water shower several inches in diameter, which fell from a height of ten to twenty feet. Publicity from four lawsuits brought against him only contributed to the spread of hydropathy.

While hydropathy was developing in Austria, Sylvester Graham (1794-1851), the acknowledged founder of Natural Hygiene and originator of the graham cracker, trained to become an evangelist in the United States. He was ordained as a Presbyterian minister in his early thirties. In 1830, he became a spokesperson for the Pennsylvania Temperance Society. Graham guaranteed that his regimen could ward off cholera, which at the time threatened to spread from Europe to America. For the following nine years he remained in great demand as a health lecturer. Cholera is an infectious disease characterized by diarrhea and cramps. In *Crusaders for Fitness: The History of American Health Reformers* (1982), Professor James C. Whorton writes: "Graham's insistence on water as the only suitable beverage was, of course, unfortunate in an epidemic of cholera, for the disease was being spread most effectively through contaminated water supplies; cheap, germicidal bourbon would have been a far safer drink."

Graham passionately posited as necessary for "salvation" abstention from: (1) intake of meat, salt, spices, and any beverage more stimulating than water; (2) "overstimulation" of the stomach, which he imagined was a "vital power" plant; (3) smoking; and (4) masturbation ("self-pollution") and sexual "excess." He warned of "eternal consequences." Consumption of flesh, he taught, provoked fleshly desire. He considered all medicines evil and regarded the frequency of nocturnal emissions as a barometer of debility (the fewer, the better). Brown (whole-wheat) bread was to Graham what brown rice was to macrobiotics founder George Ohsawa. He insisted that it be homemade from grain grown on the family farm. (His wife, not surprisingly, dissented from his dietary restrictions.) Modern "organic" farming probably would not have passed muster with Graham, who decried the use of animal-manure fertilizer as "artificially stimulating" and contributing to "debauchment" of the soil.

In *Alternative Medicine and American Religious Life* (1989), philosophy professor Robert C. Fuller traces the characteristically American belief that physical well-being depends upon an individual's cosmic rapport. He writes that Sylvester Graham "represents something of a case study in the confluence of religious intentions and health reform during the first half of the nineteenth century. . . . His ideas were so avidly appropriated by those espousing Thomsonianism [a form of herbalism], homeopathy, hydropathy, and mesmerism that they can scarcely be separated from the nineteenth century's legacy to countervailing medical traditions."

Ironically, Graham retired from public life by 1840 because of intractable bodily weakness, and consumed both meat and alcoholic beverages before his death at the age of fifty-seven. What effect, if any, his consumption of meat had upon his sex life, if any, is not recorded.

Hydropathy was introduced in the United States after the end of Graham's public career. Practitioners believed that water had the power to restore humans to a condition of purity. One of its leading figures, and an acknowledged pioneer of Natural Hygiene, was Russell Thacker Trall, M.D. (1812-1877), an institutional practitioner who combined hydropathy and puritanical Grahamism to form "Hygeio-Therapy"—"curing" by cleanliness, diet, exercise, air, and other common measures.

The hydropathy movement reached its peak around 1850 and nearly disappeared after Trall's death. But it was revived later in the century by Bavarian priest and charity-worker Sebastian Kneipp (1821-1897), author of *My Water Cure*, who combined hydropathy with herbalism. Father Kneipp's countryman, Benedict Lust (1872-1945), emigrated to the United States in 1892 and eventually acquired degrees in naturopathy, osteopathy, chiropractic, and medicine. A satisfied former patient of Kneipp's, Lust opened the Kneipp Water-Cure Institute in Brooklyn in 1895 and America's first "health food" store in 1896. In 1900, a committee of Kneipp practitioners met in the United States and decided to broaden their practice to include all "natural" modalities, and hygeiotherapy became naturopathy. In short order, Lust established in New York City the first naturopathic college—the American School of Naturopathy. Its site was shared by two other schools he operated: the New York School of Massage and the American School of Chiropractic.

Osteopathic therapy predates chiropractic. Although osteopathy is now a legitimate medical discipline in the United States, its founder, Andrew Taylor Still—who grew up in a milieu in which supposed possession by the "Holy Spirit" was commonplace—claimed that osteopathy had been revealed to him by God. He taught that the body's "life force" would create health if structural defects are removed.

Naturopathy: A Vitalistic Grab Bag

Although naturopathy did not spring from a unified doctrine and is poorly organized in both theory and practice, naturopaths generally agree that a "life force" flows through the body in various channels, and that blockages cause "imbalances" leading to disease. In *The Complete Natural-Health Consultant* (1987), naturopath Michael Van Straten notes that the "life force" concept is fundamental to naturopathy, and records the naturopathic belief that "disease is not an external invasion of bacteria or viruses but an expression of the body's healing properties at work." Van Straten further writes: "In the treatment of chronic disorders, signifying a deeper level of dysfunction, naturopaths try to stimulate the more active phase of disease and this is why naturopathic treatment at first sometimes seems to aggravate the condition before it cures it."

"The naturopath's basic argument," according to Brian Inglis in *Fringe Medicine* (1964), "is that if the body is nourished only with ingredients that it needs, and if ingredients that are inessential and harmful are so far as possible excluded, diseases can be avoided." The argument further maintains, Inglis continues, that if a disease takes hold, the body can ordinarily heal itself without the aid of drugs or surgery.

There are only two colleges of naturopathy in the United States that approach *superficial* respectability: Bastyr College in Seattle, Washington, and the National College of Naturopathic Medicine (NCNM) in Portland, Oregon. Bastyr was founded by three NCNM graduates in 1978. Its N.D. program is accredited. In addition, Bastyr has a B.S. degree program in Natural Health Sciences with majors in nutrition and Oriental medicine, and M.S. degree programs in nutrition and acupuncture. NCNM was founded in 1956. It is not accredited, but is a "Candidate for Accreditation" with the Council on Naturopathic Medical Education (CNME). The CNME is officially recognized only by a few states. However, in May 1991, the National Advisory Committee on Accreditation and Eligibility of the U.S. Department of Education voted to extend federal recognition of the CNME for three more years. The National Council Against Health Fraud responded: "This action should serve as a warning that the accreditation process is defective at its core. . . . Many will be shocked to learn that no health care guild is legally required to be scientific."

Naturopathic licensing laws exist in only seven states and the District of Columbia. Several other states have laws that permit them to practice. But in other states they are not officially allowed to do so. A directory in the January/February 1992 issue of *East West Natural Health* lists nearly four hundred naturopaths with practices in twenty-seven states, the District of Columbia, and Puerto Rico. Like Natural Hygienists, many naturopaths oppose vaccinations. One apparently nostalgic naturopath is quoted in the September 1981 issue of *Pediatrics*:

> [Vaccinations] are not known to give life-time protection, whereas actually contracting the disease does. In the old days, they used to have a "measles party" in order to deliberately expose children. I would like to see the Public Health Department make this kind of exposure available.

The Abunda Life Health Hotel and Clinic in Asbury Park, New Jersey, serves as an illustration of naturopathy. The "Abunda Life Creed" describes the body as the "temple of God," and disease as the result of "broken law." It further states: "The health we enjoy is always in direct proportion with our compliance with God's command to 'cleanse ourselves.'" According to a brochure, services and features include a "Thermogenic Fat Burning and Internal Purification Room" for burning excess body fat (which admittedly "looks like a sauna"), a "non-burn" ultraviolet Sun Studio, "medical hypnotherapy," colon hydrotherapy, aromatherapy, laughter therapy, foot reflexology, skin brushing, massage, iridology evaluation, career aptitude testing, "life force testing," Bible study, "C.M." (Christian meditation), and spiritual healing. The brochure brushes dietitians aside as lackeys of the medical establishment whose sole function is to plan institutional menus.

According to the January 1992 issue of Abunda Life's journal, *The Abundant Life Times*, the Thermogenic Fat Burning Room does more than burn body fat; it also "internally purifies deeply stored poisons accumulated over a lifetime." "Thermogenic" treatments are priced at $35.

Unlike Natural Hygienists, not all naturopaths subscribe to vegetarianism. For example, in *Traditional Foods Are Your Best Medicine* (1987), licensed naturopath Ronald F. Schmid, who worked as a "nutritional consultant" under the direction of FAIM trustee Michael Schachter, M.D. (see Chapter 7), advocates a diet composed of equal proportions of: (1) animal-source foods; (2) raw greens and sprouts; and (3) whole grains, other vegetables, and fruits.

Re-Animator

The revitalizing role that Kneipp served with respect to hydropathy, Herbert M. Shelton (1895-1985) assumed with respect to Russell Trall's hygeiotherapy, which evolved into Natural Hygiene.

In a 1978 issue of *Health Science*, published by the American Natural Hygiene Society, Shelton described his educational background. At the age of sixteen, having undergone "the usual brainwashing process of the public school system in Greenville, Texas," he "revolted against the whole political, religious, medical, and social system." After serving in the Army during World War I, he received his first degree, that of "Doctor of Physiological Therapeutics," from the Macfadden College of Physcultopathy. Later called the International College of Drugless Physicians, this school had been established in 1913 by the self-proclaimed "father of physical culture," bodybuilder Bernarr Macfadden (1868-1955). The cover of each issue of Macfadden's popular magazine *Physical Culture* bore the legend: "Weakness is a Crime; don't be a Criminal." Throughout his life, Macfadden slept on the floor. Although he departed from Grahamism in championing sexual indulgence, Macfadden is perhaps not best known for having invented the "peniscope," an electrical penis enlarger.

Next, Shelton took a postgraduate course at the Lindlahr College of Natural Therapeutics in Chicago. Henry Lindlahr, M.D., was a proponent of iridology. In *A Doctor's Views on Nature Care*, he professed that: (1) "there is . . . a morality of the physical as well as of the spiritual"; (2) "all that which we call disease, suffering or evil are due to violations of Nature's laws and . . . consequently the only possible permanent cure lies in a return to Nature"; and (3) "all disease is caused by something that interferes with, diminishes or disturbs the normal inflow and distribution of vital energy throughout the system."

From Chicago, Shelton went to New York, where, "after nine months of brainwashing," he received doctoral degrees from schools founded by Benedict Lust, one in naturopathy and the other in chiropractic. Then he returned to Chicago to do postgraduate work at another chiropractic college, which was "accompanied and succeeded by thirty-one months of apprenticeship in four different institutions, where the most valuable thing I learned was what not to do."

Shelton said he had "confused Natural Hygiene with what was called Nature Cure" (a transitional form of naturopathy centered on hydropathy). He credited Sylvester Graham and Russell Thacker Trall with having had the greatest influence on his early thinking. The first of his approximately forty books, *Fundamentals of Nature Cure*, was published in 1920. In his "magnum opus," *Human Life: Its Philosophy and Laws*, published in 1928, Shelton's fourteen "commandments" for correct living include: getting "as much sunshine as possible"; marriage, homemaking, and child-rearing; and avoidance of sexual "excess." In the same year, he opened Dr. Shelton's Health School in San Antonio, Texas, which operated at seven different locations until 1981. Its aim was to teach "students and guests to build health with the causes of health and to cease relying on the practices of traditional medicine." From 1934 to 1941, Shelton produced a seven-volume series called *The Hygienic System*. In 1941 he launched *Dr. Shelton's Hygienic Review*, a monthly magazine that was published for about forty years.

In 1982, a federal court jury awarded $873,000 to the survivors of William Carlton, a forty-nine-year-old man who had died after undergoing a distilled-water fast for thirty days at Shelton's Health School. An article in the *Los Angeles Daily Journal* stated that Carlton had died of bronchial pneumonia resulting from a weakened condition in which he lost fifty pounds during the last month of his life. The article also noted that he was the sixth person in five years who had died while undergoing "treatment" at the school. Shelton and his associate, chiropractor Vivian V. Vetrano, claimed in their appeal that Carlton had persisted in fasting after Vetrano had advised him to stop. However, the verdict was upheld by the Fifth Circuit Court of Appeals, and the U.S. Supreme Court declined further review.

Graham's Legacy

The fountainhead of today's Natural Hygiene activity, the American Natural Hygiene Society (ANHS), was founded in 1948 by Shelton and several associates. Something of an anachronistic reincarnation of the American Physiological Society, organized by Graham and Trall a century earlier, the ANHS has its headquarters in Tampa, Florida. Regular ANHS membership costs $25 and includes a subscription to *Health Science*. The treasurer's report for 1991 lists an income of $526,532 and states that the group had over 6,700 members. However, since the listed total of membership dues was $101,857, the actual number of members may have been about four thousand. The ANHS has actively promoted certification of "organic" foods and vigorously opposed compulsory immunization and food irradiation.

In the above-mentioned 1978 interview, Shelton stated that he had "about concluded that more professional *Hygienists* is not a worthwhile goal," that "an army of [nonprofessional] *Hygienists* will eliminate the need for the professionals," and that the ANHS "should bend every effort to prevent it from being monopolized by professionals." He further stated that the ANHS should "expend [its] energy . . . in making new *Hygienists* from raw material [rather] than to expend its resources to unbrainwash members of the treating cults. . . . Once a therapist always a therapist." Nevertheless, each issue of *Health Science* contains, "as a public service," a Professional Referral List of members of the International Association of Professional Natural Hygienists. The November/December 1992 list contains thirty-two names. Most are chiropractors, but a few hold a medical, osteopathic, or naturopathic degree. The list includes twelve "certified" and eight "associate" members in the United States, and others located in Australia, Canada, England, Greece, Israel, Japan, and Poland. Certified members include ANHS founders and "subsequent members who have successfully completed an internship (or its equivalent) in Natural Hygiene care with an emphasis on Fasting Supervision."

Back to School: High School Dropout Becomes "College" Administrator

Grassroots Natural Hygienist T.C. Fry was born near Bennington, Oklahoma, in 1926. According to the cover of his paperback *Laugh Your Way to Health* (1991):

> Mr. Fry's quest for reality began before six years of age. He was raised a fundamentalist Christian in what was variously called the Holiness Church or Pentecostal Church. There was public confession, rolling in the aisles by women and several baptismal rites

every summer. With the orientation in these churches, he believed in the presence of both God and Satan. He sought them on a personal basis at that age.

Mr. Fry never completed high school. He went to college on passing a college entrance examination. He dropped out of college within three months "because they had nothing of significance to teach."

At age 16, Mr. Fry ran away from home and has been economically independent since. Until his marriage at age 26 he spent most of his time in libraries. Pursuing a business career since then, Mr. Fry has traveled over much of the world and acquired a large private library of books.

In the mid-1970s, Fry began using the term "Life Science" to denote Natural Hygiene. In *Program for Dynamic Health: An Introduction to Natural Hygiene*, published by ANHS in 1974, he paid tribute to Shelton for having steered him, via the book *Superior Nutrition*, onto "a completely living food diet." Before starting this diet, Fry had weighed about 197 pounds at a height of 5 feet 6½ inches. Clad in bathing-briefs and striking bodybuilder poses, Fry appears in "after" photos on the paperback's cover. Inside, he describes how and why he forgoes using soap, toothbrushes, toothpaste, and shaving cream.

In 1982, Fry founded a correspondence school called the College of Health Science in Austin, Texas. It had three names before evolving into the Life Science Institute (LSI) in 1983. Adoption of this last name was prompted by the objection of the district attorney's office to Fry's unauthorized use of the word "college" in the school's letterhead. Harvey Diamond, co-author of *Fit for Life* (1985) and *Living Health* (1987), received his "Ph.D. in nutritional science" from Fry's unaccredited school in February 1983. His wife, co-author Marilyn, holds a "master's degree" from the school. Both appeared on ABC News' "Nightline" in 1986. In defense of his "doctorate," Harvey claimed that the "University of Paris School of Medicine" was then teaching Fry's course to 5,500 medical students.

In 1987, my colleague Ira Milner, R.D., phoned the French consulate to obtain this school's address. He discovered that it had at least a dozen locations. So Milner called Fry, who said his course was taught at Bobigny. Milner wrote to Bobigny several times. Finally, in a letter dated November 19, 1987, the director of the University of Paris Medical School stated that the administration had never heard of either Fry or his "so-called" college. The director disclosed that the school did offer a course in "Natural Medicine." But he described it as an experimental and somewhat contradictory elective, not leading to any certification whatsoever. Moreover, he stated that the total number of medical students was only 800.

In a letter addressed to Milner dated February 22, 1988, however, Fry claimed he was an "honorary professor" at the University of Paris and that he lectured there occasionally. He stated that 1,200 nursing and medical students there take his course, and that graduates receive a "certificate called Dr. of Nurturotherapy [sic]."

In 1986, LSI was put out of business temporarily when the State of Texas finally barred "Professor" Fry by permanent injunction from representing his operation as a college and from granting either degrees or academic credits without state certification. The school's 1987-1988 Student Directory lists over 2,000 names and addresses. According to the October 1989 issue of LSI's magazine, *Healthful Living*, the school had been padlocked for two months by the IRS for nonpayment of back taxes. Later that year, I enrolled. A doctorate, alas, did not await me—just a voluminous correspondence course of 150 lessons detailing Fry's vituperative views. It supposedly required about a year to complete, and cost $1,475. LSI's description of the course carried the promise: "Upon successful completion of this course, you'll be uniquely qualified to practice this science so that nearly 100% of your clients will overcome their problems, be rejuvenated and live at a high level of health." Lessons cover the legal, managerial, and marketing aspects of nutrition counseling.

LSI again foundered in October 1990, when Fry, age 64, was arrested and his home and office were searched. The charge was, in his own words, that of "injury to an elderly person"—a "guest" undergoing "Hygienic" care. But in the summer of 1991 the school assumed the name Health Excellence Systems (HES). HES offered a "Basic Course in the Nutritional, Behavioral and Health Sciences" consisting of twenty-six lessons for $227.50, optional certification as a "Health Specialist" for an additional $75 (available to students who pass an "extensive" exam covering the twenty-six lessons), and a "Master Course" consisting of over 130 lessons. In a section titled "You Can Become an Expert Nutritionist in Less Than a Year!" the brochure asks: "Can you imagine learning and understanding more about nutrition than so-called nutritionists know after going through college, much special training, and many years of practice in the field?" The brochure further states that "diseases are not caused by germs or viruses" but by malnutrition and "toxicosis." The American Health Sciences Institute emerged later in 1991. It is "affiliated" with HES, has the same address, and offers the same course at a prepayment cost of $1,475. There are no admission prerequisites and the one-page application is easy to complete. A 1992 ad for the institute states: "Even if those who consult you are suffering from 'incurable' diseases, you can teach them to discontinue easily recognizable causes and to adopt the elements of health. Diseases disappear very quickly when causes are removed and the needs of life are appropriately met."

"I Live on Fruit"

In a pamphlet entitled "The Great AIDS Hoax," Fry flatly discounts the viral etiology of AIDS, and instead blames "drugs and other poisons." He further claims that discontinuation of the intake of such substances will result in "the highest level of health possible." Fry excels at oversimplification, advocating fruitarianism and virtually unlimited exposure to sunlight. He is the co-author of *I Live on Fruit* (1990), which supposedly presents "proof that the fruitarian diet is not only nutritionally adequate in every respect, but is actually superior to any and all other foods humans may eat!" In the October 1989 *Healthful Living*, he states that fruits "furnish our every nutrient need," that they are "the only complete food which, in themselves, meet our nutritive requirements." In the "Health in the News" department of that same issue, the idea of skin cancer resulting from overexposure to sunlight is roundly repudiated: "If sunshine is bad, why should there be several times as many acute illnesses in the winter when there's little sunshine as in the summer when there is much?" The item concludes: "If you want to follow a healthful course, do just the opposite to what medical minds advise."

In a letter to Fry printed in the October 1990 issue, an LSI student living in England expressed her "urgent" concern over whether fruits alone constitute a "balanced diet." She reported that: (1) both of her children, ages twenty months and four years, had vomited in response to the consumption of nuts, and "will eat only fruit"; (2) the family's diet consists "basically" of oranges, apples, bananas, pears, grapes, apricots, kiwis, dates, black currants, and yellow raisins; (3) she is twenty-five years old and 5'6" tall, weighs 100 pounds, and feels cold in the summer; and (4) her husband is twenty-seven years old and 5'8" tall, weighs 112 pounds, and "looks terrible." "We both would like to gain weight," she said. Fry replied that: (1) "Nuts are not necessary for children or anyone else"; (2) the mother had erred in combining "two digestively incompatible ingredients"—nuts and honey—in making "nutmilk" for her son; (3) fruits contain all that her children require "proportionally to their needs including

amino acids averaging about 1% . . . the same as has mother's milk"; and
(4) her coldness may be the result of intense "detoxifying processes." He
advised her: (1) against listening to nutritionists, friends, and neighbors;
(2) to eat dried fruits when she feels cold; and (3) to perform weightlifting,
pushups, and other exercises to gain weight. Fry further told the student she
was fortunate to have a "hygienic" husband.

The style of present-day Hygienic gurus betrays a resemblance to
Sylvester Graham's religiosity. In a December 1989 letter to me, Fry
related how he teaches the many Christians he works with about Natural
Hygiene: "Put only God-made foods into your body. If man did anything
at all with it, even if only heating, don't eat it." He further stated that he
holds "a dramatic response to be worth thousands of words of explanation." A 1992 newsletter published by a grassroots Hygienic enterprise in
Mt. Vernon, Washington, called "Get Well/Stay Well, America!" features
information on the Christian Natural Hygiene Association, books titled
Christ the Healer and *Why Christians Get Sick*, and an audiocassette album
titled "God's Guidelines to Radiant Health." It states:

> Our America was founded as a Christian Nation in 1607. Natural
> Hygiene began as Christian Health Revolution in 1822. Let us
> revive these old-time values of God, Health, and Country in the
> 1990s!

Fasting for All

"Therapeutic" is something of a dirty word for Natural Hygienists. According to an ANHS brochure:

> A thoroughgoing rest, which includes fasting, is the most favor-
> able condition under which an ailing body can purify and repair
> itself. Fasting is the total abstinence from all liquid and solid foods
> except distilled water. During a fast the body's recuperative forces
> are marshaled and all of its energies are directed toward the
> recharging of the nervous system, the elimination of toxic accumu-
> lations, and the repair and rejuvenation of tissue. Stored within
> each organism's tissues are nutrient reserves which it will use to
> carry on metabolism and repair work. Until these reserves are
> depleted, no destruction of healthy tissue or "starvation" can
> occur.

ANHS publications promote fasting for children as well as for adults. The
brochure also states:

Natural Hygiene rejects the use of medications, blood transfusions, radiation, dietary supplements, and any other means employed to treat or "cure" various ailments. These therapies interfere with or destroy vital processes and tissue. Recovery from disease takes place in spite of, and not because of, the drugging and "curing" practices.

Natural Hygiene is contrasted with macrobiotics in a 1984 issue of ANHS's journal: "Unlike Natural Hygiene, which bases its system upon a profound respect for *Nature* and the inherent power and intelligence of the human organism, Macrobiotics remains content to experiment with the age-old belief in human *domination* of nature."

"Food Combining"

Like macrobiotics, Natural Hygiene conspicuously incorporates a system of "food combining." However, the Hygienic system is somewhat more clear-cut and more patently pseudoscientific than that of macrobiotics. In *Food Combining Made Easy*—a "nutrition classic," its cover would have us believe—Shelton wrote:

> To a single article of food that is a starch-protein combination, the body can easily adjust its juices. . . to the digestive requirements of the food. But when two foods are eaten with different . . . digestive needs, this precise adjustment of juices to requirements becomes impossible.

Natural Hygienists believe, for example, that consuming a high-protein food and a high-carbohydrate food at the same meal will, at the least, tax the body's enzymatic capacity.

Such pronouncements were debunked more than fifty years ago in both scientific and popular literature, but the Hygienic faithful still hold them dear. In a review of studies of human gastric digestion of proteins and carbohydrates in health and disease, published in 1934 in the *Journal of the American Medical Association*, researcher Martin E. Rehfuss, M.D., presented detailed evidence that "clearly proves that any presumed incompatibility between protein and carbohydrate food . . . is certainly not sustained." Of the likes of Shelton, Rehfuss wrote: "One searches in vain through the literature revealing several thousand contributions by research workers on diet and nutrition to find any real scientific work by these reformers."

In *Food Combining*, Shelton grouped foods "according to their composition and sources of origin": (1) "proteins," including nuts, peanuts, and avocados; (2) "starches" and sweet fruits, including peanuts (again), chestnuts, pumpkin, bananas, and mangoes; (3) "fats," including most nuts (again) and avocados (again); (4) "acid fruits," including citrus fruit and tomatoes; (5) "sub-acid" fruits, including pears and apricots; (6) non-starchy and green vegetables, including lettuce, broccoli, and watercress; and (7) melons, including watermelon, honeydew, and cantaloupe. Hygienic classification schemes differ somewhat, but certain listed foods, such as garlic (an "irritant"), and all animal-source foods, are not recommended under any circumstances.

Shelton taught that certain combinations are indigestible: (1) "acids" and starches, (2) proteins and starches, (3) acids and proteins, (4) fats and proteins, (5) sugars and proteins, (6) sugars and starches (note that Shelton classified sweet fruits with starches), (7) melons and anything other than fresh fruit, and (8) even two different proteins.

Despite a plethora of absurdities, Natural Hygiene has enjoyed a renaissance in recent years with the Diamond's *Fit for Life* and *Living Health*, Judy Mazel's *Beverly Hills Diet* (1979) and *Beverly Hills Lifetime Diet Plan* (1982), and Anthony Robbins' *Unlimited Power* (1986).

The 1990 Conference

Both Harvey Diamond and T.C. Fry were present at the American Natural Hygiene Society's 42nd Annual International Natural Living Conference, held at Hofstra University for five days in the summer of 1990. I attended the morning and afternoon sessions on July 28 and found a revivalist atmosphere and about 250 people present. One person sitting near me in the first row insisted mysteriously that Hygiene "changes you." I didn't pursue the subject.

Ronald G. Cridland, M.D., director of the Fundamental Health Center in Toronto, Canada, was the first speaker of the day. His topic was "Natural Hygiene: The Science of Health." Cridland referred to Greek mythology and great medical reformers such as Ignaz Semmelweis and Louis Pasteur in an effort to lend credence and historical depth to the work of Graham, Shelton, and other Hygienic pioneers. He eulogized Semmelweis as a man who "did everything he could to try and raise the education of his peers. He gave lectures, and he wrote papers . . . and he was always put down. In fact, eventually he died insane . . . a couple of hundred years before his time." Cridland then trivialized the practice of immunization.

He summed up Hygienic philosophy: "Disease is a result of a susceptible organism, because you are not living within your capacity. . . . The idea is to identify and remove factors that interfere with the healing process in our diet, in our environment, in our activity, and in our psychology." "Raw vegetables," he said, "probably should provide the majority of your diet." He added: "At one time we may have been designed to subsist largely on fruits, because fruits were more like vegetables than they are today. They had less sugar content, more fiber content."

When Cridland was finished, the moderator instructed us to turn to the persons next to us and hug them twice.

The next speaker was Alec Burton, M.Sc., D.O., D.C., director of the Hygeia Health Institute in Sydney, Australia. His lecture was titled "Diet and Nutrition from the Natural Hygiene Perspective." Burton likened extracted oils to sugar, stated that "no fat or oil should be added to food in any way at all," and described processed fats as "highly dangerous." He claimed (incorrectly) that the National Research Council "recommends one percent of calories from fat . . . about thirty calories or . . . the equivalent of half a teaspoon of oil. And that's what they recommend as probably the ideal."

Taking aim at what he considered the follies of nutritional science, Burton said that "the history of nutrition . . . often reads like the work of a mentally defective person on a bad day." He cited the mistaking of beriberi for an infection and a commission's conclusion that pellagra was caused by the bite of a horsefly. "I want to go on," he said. "There are endless stories associated with very, very serious errors and serious mistakes."

Burton suggested that the need for protein is about 20 grams a day, and warned against eating polar bear liver (which is extremely high in vitamin A). Unlike macrobiotic adherents, he boasted, Natural Hygienists do not develop scurvy. But later he advised against eating too much fruit. Burton ended his talk with the pseudoscientific telltale: "Really good science is also good common sense."

He was followed by chiropractor Ralph Cinque, director of the Hygeia Health Retreat in Yorktown, Texas, whose topic was: "Setting Your Goals as a Natural Hygienist." "More than anything else," said Cinque, "Hygiene should free you from therapeutic dependencies, both physically and psychologically. I want to remind people of something: that there is a veritable army of therapists out there waiting like sharks to justify giving you treatments. And I believe that the best attitude that you can have is to be skeptical of all of it. . . . And I believe that the extent to which you can be free of therapeutic dependencies should be the measure of your success as a Hygienist."

"Blind Faith"

As I sought the dining room at lunchtime, a gentleman engaged me in conversation and introduced me to his daughter. They had come to the conference from the Midwest. His daughter, he said, had been diagnosed with chronic fatigue syndrome (CFS). No form of therapy has been proven effective against CFS, but unproven therapies abound.

I interviewed both father and daughter and obtained a diet history from the daughter. She was twenty-two years old and weighed between ninety-eight and one hundred pounds at a height of 5'5". Based on an assumed small body frame type, her weight was at least 11 percent below a desirable weight of 113 pounds. At this weight, any ambulatory woman of her age not suffering from starvation would require an average daily intake of at least 1,675 kilocalories just to prevent weight loss. The typical food intake she reported suggested that this need was not being met. It consisted of melons for breakfast; two bananas and three peaches for lunch; a salad of Romaine lettuce, carrots, zucchini, avocado, and tomato— without dressing—for dinner; and water between meals. She had recently undergone a medically supervised distilled-water fast for eighteen days.

Her father explained: "We went all over the country looking for a cure, and there is no cure for it." Many drugs had been considered, he said, "but drugs have such a significant adverse effect." Her condition had improved somewhat in the course of a month she'd spent in the care of a conventional physician in California. Nevertheless, they'd gone to Denver to consult an uncredentialed "natural healer" who reputedly had worked with rock stars, using diet, "mental control," exercise, and relaxation to maintain their "high energy level." At that point, his daughter had felt so bad "she could hardly get up in the morning. . . . She couldn't go to college." She had been, her father tellingly summed up, "very depressed." Using *Fit for Life* as a guide, the so-called healer had worked with her five days a week for six weeks, two years earlier. But for about a year and a half, she had been following a stricter Hygienic regimen. Now she was teetering on the brink of emaciation. "We went on blind faith," her father conceded.

Keeping the Faith

Lunch consisted of raw, fresh, nonstarchy vegetables, fresh fruit, and raw almonds. As we neared the end of a long buffet, I expressed my concern that no dressing would be available. But, in fact, there were two dressings, of a sort—one a thick, bland avocado dip; the other like watered-down, unsweetened punch. I did not enjoy lunch.

The next lecturer was Jim Lennon, executive director of ANHS and a former musician. Jim offered "faith-keeping" tactics to ward off inquiries by well-meaning but "misguided" significant others into the safety and wherefores of Hygienic eating, and then gave a pep talk.

"What is the famous question?" he asked. "Right: 'Where do you get the protein?' The answer is, 'It's in everything! Thanks for asking; how are the kids?'" Why should one be curt? "Because you don't want to talk about that, do you? . . . You can change the subject. You are not working for the other people that you run into in your life. You don't have to answer every question. You don't have to be a physiologist."

He told us we were leaders and celebrities because we "don't go along with the crowd." We were "different," he said; we had the courage to go our own way. "How unique that is!"

"Who bothers you?" he asked. "The answer is, the people who know they should be doing it. . . . As soon as someone starts bothering you, that's a victory. . . . They're trying to figure out a way to make it okay that they don't [follow the diet]." Later, Lennon stated that grandparents "can only inspire" dietarily recalcitrant grandchildren.

The last afternoon speaker, chiropractor D.J. Scott, restated Lennon's sentiments toward doubters of Natural Hygiene: "You start out with the realization that people challenge you because . . . somehow or other they feel a wee bit threatened." Scott declared that Hygienists do not need such procedures as hysterectomies and prostate surgery. "I have seen massive tumors of the pelvic organs, women with thyroid tumors as large as a seven-month pregnancy, ovarian cysts that completely fill up an abdomen. And these things," he said, despite being long-standing conditions tempting immediate surgery, "do gradually diminish, not in one week of fasting, not in a month of fasting, but over months of Hygienic living."

Throughout the program, there was considerable talk of vitality. Yet, in just the vicinity of my seat, I counted thirteen people who had their eyes closed and appeared to be napping.

Neither Natural Nor Hygienic

In *Science and Unreason* (1982), Daisie and Michael Radner put forth the "marks of pseudoscience," which include: (1) wholesale rehabilitation of a disproved theory for moral or pragmatic reasons; (2) "playing another ball game"—nonadherence to the accepted principles and procedures that constitute the scientific method; (3) invocation of myths; (4) selection and organization of data so as to conform to a particular bias; (5) an exegetic or esoteric approach to the scientific literature—a misapprehension of science as "all statements by scientists, open to interpretation"; and (6) refusal to revise a theory in the light of criticism. The authors suggest that just one of these characteristics is sufficient to render a theory or practice pseudoscientific. Natural Hygiene exhibits all six of the above marks.

As humans are by nature omnivorous, having eaten meat for at least 4.5 million years since achieving their first semblance of humanity, the practice of Natural Hygiene cannot rightly be called natural. The authors of *The Paleolithic Prescription* (1988) recommend that usage of the word "natural" be restricted to the meaning: "in accord with our genetically determined biochemistry and physiology." Natural Hygiene is not in such accord.

Neither is it hygienic—that is, likely to promote or preserve health. Any philosophy that trivializes nutrient needs, encourages prolonged fasting, and discourages medical interventions almost across the board—as Natural Hygiene does—is not likely to benefit health if followed rigidly. For one thing, Hygiene's proscription of both dairy products and supplements in the context of its primarily raw-food diet is an invitation to osteoporosis.

Fortunately, Hygienic dietary guidelines vary, and adherents vary considerably in the extent to which they follow them. For example, in *Fit for Life*, the Diamonds reluctantly make allowance for the consumption of milk (preferably unpasteurized) and plain yogurt, and their dinner menus include seafood and fowl. And in a *Health Science* interview, Ralph Cinque conceded that people should not be made to "suffer mental distress over their food combinations."

The Bottom Line

No scientific study has ever compared the morbidity and mortality of Hygienists with those of non-Hygienists. But it seems to me that the hazards of Natural Hygiene significantly outweigh the possible benefits.

5

"Esoteric Stuff":
The Edgar Cayce Tradition

The "Outer Limits"

Born in 1877, alleged clairvoyant Edgar Cayce was dubbed the "Sleeping Prophet" by his biographer Jess Stern. A harbinger of "New Age" trance channeling, Cayce gave well over 14,000 "psychic readings" between 1910 and early 1945, when he died of a massive stroke. He was born and raised on a tobacco farm near Hopkinsville, Kentucky, in the small, isolated, rural community of Christian County. In *Edgar Cayce on Diet and Health* (1969), his son, Hugh Lynn Cayce (1907-1982), wrote:

> At the age of six or seven, he told his parents that he was able to see and talk to "visions,'" sometimes of relatives who had recently died. His parents attributed this to the overactive imagination of a lonely child who had been influenced by the dramatic language of the revival meetings which were popular in that section of the country.

Nonphysical beings are said to have been Cayce's childhood companions. In the introduction to *Edgar Cayce Speaks* (1969), Cayce is described as a child who was "troubled" and rather "backward," constantly seeking solace and refuge in the Bible under the influence of his devoutly religious mother. His alleged talent for healing first appeared when he was sixteen years old. Time-Life Books' *Powers of Healing* describes the event:

> Young Cayce had been struck at the base of the spine by a pitched

63

ball, and although he sustained no serious injury, he began behaving somewhat strangely. At home that evening the normally docile Edgar stormed about, shouting, laughing uproariously, throwing things, and quarreling with everyone. His father sent him to bed, where the boy soon fell into a profound sleep. As his concerned parents stood over him, a voice seemingly brought up from the depths of Edgar's body commanded Mrs. Cayce to prepare a special poultice and to place it on the back of his head. The boy then slept normally, and the next morning he arose his old self again, with no apparent recollection of the strange happenings of the previous evening.

In 1898, at age twenty-one, Cayce suffered from a chronically hoarse throat and intermittent laryngitis. He was a salesman for a wholesale stationery company, but his affliction resisted medical treatment and obliged him to give up his occupation. In desperation, he consulted a hypnotist, who provided temporary relief. Another hypnotist asked him to describe, while he was in a trance, the cause of his ailment and its cure. Cayce supposedly did so, and it is said that at the end of the session his voice was normal. This "cure," however, was not permanent.

The hypnotist proposed that Cayce use this method to render diagnoses for others, and in 1901 he began doing so, entering a trance and offering guidance to persons who were present or who had mailed a request for service. His earlier readings were given with the assistance of osteopaths and homeopaths, and his diagnoses and prescriptions reflect this association. He often diagnosed spinal lesions as the source of pain, and prescribed spinal manipulation. In *A Seer Out of Season: The Life of Edgar Cayce* (1989), Harmon Hartzell Bro, Ph.D., indicates that Cayce "regularly required" the presence of a physician in order to give a "full-fledged" reading.

In 1902 he took a clerical position in a bookstore, but within a few years he left the store, became a photographer, and opened his own studio. This was destroyed by two fires. With the publication of a two-page article on him in the *New York Times* in 1910, Edgar Cayce—a Sunday school teacher who had received no education beyond the ninth grade—gained nationwide renown. In 1912 he opened a new photographic studio and, according to his son Hugh Lynn, "attempted to stop" giving readings. This studio also burned, and the business went bankrupt. But, as news of his "healings" spread, thousands sought his help. After entering a self-induced hypnotic state, he would prescribe dietary and other remedies, advise clients on reincarnation and the occult, and practice prognostication.

In the early 1920s, Cayce changed his trade to that of a full-time psychic, for which purpose he had an office and a business card identifying him as a "psychic diagnostician." According to *Harper's Encyclopedia of Mystical and Paranormal Experience* (1991), Cayce's diagnoses were based on a variety of causative factors, including glandular conditions, childhood bumps and bruises ("which produced lesions that later caused disturbances"), and karmic conditions ("spiritual heredity"). In *Flim-Flam!* (1987), professional magician James Randi notes that Cayce "even gave diagnoses when the 'patients' were *dead!* . . . Surely, death is a very serious symptom and should be detectable."

Although *The Aquarian Guide to the New Age* (1990) characterizes Cayce as a "somewhat" fundamentalist Christian, his "entranced" personality was that of a Theosophist of sorts (see Chapter 8). According to his readings, his "past lives" included those of a "celestial being," an Atlantean, an Egyptian high priest, a Persian ruler, a Trojan warrior, and a minor disciple of Christ. His "revelations," such as those on the so-called lost years of Jesus Christ, were allegedly derived from our "collective consciousness" rather than from particular spirits. The failure of mythical Atlantis to resurface in the late 1960s is but one of a score of wrong predictions. In the 1930s, Cayce prophesied that the Second Coming of Christ would occur in 1998. In 1941, he predicted that land would appear in both the Atlantic and the Pacific within a few years, that most of New York City would disappear within another generation, and that the southern portions of Carolina and Georgia would disappear even sooner.

In *The Outer Limits of Edgar Cayce's Power* (1971), Cayce's sons Edgar Evans and Hugh Lynn reported there were 14,246 readings on file, comprising over 50,000 single-spaced typewritten pages of stenographic transcripts—more than ten million words. (Records of readings given between 1901 and 1909 had not been preserved). They estimated that 14.4 percent of the available readings were incorrect. This percentage represents 2,051 unsuccessful readings. Cayce's sons stated that most of these unsuccessful readings pertained not to physical or psychological health, but to "miscellaneous" subjects, such as missing persons, oil wells, and buried treasure. This is not surprising given the quite objective nature of such affairs. Moreover, the so-called "85 percent accuracy record" serves as an example of wishful thinking, since it is based on a mere 150 readings, the results of half of which were not recorded.

Cayce was supposedly directed by dreams and trance readings to move to Virginia Beach, Virginia, and set up an institution of higher learning there. He fulfilled such instructions in 1928 with the establishment of a hospital and Atlantic University (chartered in 1930). But these foundered during the Great Depression and had to be closed in 1931. Cayce, Hugh Lynn, and associates wasted no time regrouping, forming the Association for Research and Enlightenment (A.R.E.) and launching the "Search for God" study-group movement that same year.

In the biographical tribute *There Is a River*, Cayce's friend Thomas Sugrue wrote:

> It is a stern set of ethics that emerges from the readings. No lukewarm embracing of theological virtues will satisfy them. They insist on perfection as the goal, and every misstep must be retraced, every injury undone, every injustice rectified. The newer, lenient interpretations of Christianity are not tolerated.

The Legacies of Edgar Cayce

Five organizations have grown up around Cayce's work. The A.R.E. headquarters, which occupies an entire city block in Virginia Beach, is home to four of them: A.R.E., Inc., the Edgar Cayce Foundation, Atlantic University, and the Harold J. Reilly School of Massotherapy. The oldest of these is Atlantic University, which opened and closed in 1931 and re-opened in 1985. The university shares both facilities and personnel with A.R.E., but has its own board of trustees. Cayce's son Charles Thomas Cayce, Ph.D., whose doctorate is in child psychology, has been acting president of the university since late 1988. Although it is unaccredited, it awards a master of arts degree in "transpersonal studies"—a term described in its catalogue as "an appropriate expression of the philosophies of the Edgar Cayce tradition." Its courses, several of which may be taken via correspondence, cover such subjects as parapsychology, dream interpretation, divination, and life after death.

The Reilly School, which operates under the auspices of Atlantic University, was founded in 1931 and reopened in 1986. Certified by the Commonwealth of Virginia, the school offers a 600-hour diploma program in massage therapy. The program includes instruction in shiatsu, foot reflexology, hydrotherapy, diet, and preventive healthcare based on the Cayce readings. The school also offers workshops on biofeedback and Cayce home remedies.

The Edgar Cayce Foundation, chartered in 1948, was formed to preserve the Cayce readings and supporting documentation.

The A.R.E. and Its Enterprises: Hope and Magic

The A.R.E. functions as an eclectic "New Age" nerve center, from which emanates a steady flow of seminars and publications. A 1991 brochure describes it as "a living network of people who are finding a deeper meaning in life through the psychic work of Edgar Cayce." In 1976, Hugh Lynn Cayce became board chairman and his son, Charles Thomas Cayce, became president. The A.R.E. headquarters, a modern three-story building in Virginia Beach, includes a visitor/conference center, a library, and the A.R.E. bookstore. It receives more than 40,000 visitors and conference attendees annually. With more than 50,000 volumes, the library has one of the world's largest collections of parapsychological and metaphysical literature. The A.R.E.'s 1988 gross income was $7.8 million, including $2.2 million from membership dues and $2.4 million from sales of educational materials. Its 1991 revenues totalled $9 million.

Standard membership costs $30 per year, but nine-month "introductory" memberships are available for $15 or $20. Members receive the bimonthly magazine *Venture Inward*. They also may borrow books from the A.R.E. Library, join a study group, and attend or send their children to A.R.E.'s summer camp in the Appalachian foothills. They are further entitled to discounts on A.R.E. conferences, and referrals to over four hundred practitioners who use the Cayce approach. Members are also invited to participate in "home research projects," in which they carry out some "psychic" activity and report the results. A 1991 issue of the *Home Research Project* bulletin states: "The main commitment of A.R.E. as a research organization is to encourage you to test concepts in the Cayce readings and to look for—and expect—results." The study groups center on such concerns as diet, the laws of reincarnation (karma), metaphysical dream interpretation, and the spiritual legacies of ancient Egypt and Atlantis. According to an A.R.E. letter: "Thousands gather together in small groups all over the country to study and apply spiritual principles in daily living." The July/August 1991 *Venture Inward* reported an A.R.E. membership of about seventy-five thousand. But a form letter from A.R.E. president Charles Thomas Cayce, dated November 27 of that year, noted a decrease in membership. In September 1992, A.R.E.'s Susan Foley informed me that membership was approximately thirty-nine thousand, plus about a thousand subscribers. *Venture Inward* includes such "news" items as "Depression breeds negative thinking" and "Yuppie values don't lead to happiness."

A.R.E. mailings to prospective members state: "There is no human problem for which the Cayce predictions do not offer hope." A.R.E. "research reports," based on the Cayce readings, are available on a wide variety of topics, including scar removal, warts, arthritis, diabetes, and multiple sclerosis.

Many of Cayce's remedies are sold through the mail by Home Health Products, Inc., also in Virginia Beach. Home Health specializes in "natural products for a holistic approach to health care" and bills itself as an "official supplier of Edgar Cayce products for health, beauty, and wellness." Its own products include skin conditioners, laxatives, and a few supplements, but its catalog also offers supplements made by other companies. Products advertised therein have included: (1) *ANF-22*, touted as "powerful relief from the pain, swelling and stiffness of arthritis"; (2) *Aphro* "Herbal Love Tonic"; (3) *Bio Ear*, said to provide "all-natural relief for ringing, buzzing, and noise in the ear"; (4) *Brain Waves*, described as a mental stimulant; (5) *Cata-Vite* (formerly *Cata-Rx*), said to be "a safe non-prescription formula which counteracts nutritional deficiencies associated with age-related cataracts"; (6) *His Ease*, alleged to "increase seminal fluid and sexual virility"; (7) *Kidney Flush*, claimed to "help flush away urinary infections"; (8) *Liva-Life*, supposed help for "toxic overload"; (9) *Liver Tonic Detoxifier*, "an all-natural mixture that detoxifies and cleanses the liver"; (10) *Prostate Plus*, proposed as an alternative to surgery; (11) *Ribo Flex*, "muscle/joint nourishment that reduces painful muscle spasms and enhances natural flexing action"; (12) *Sugar Block*, said to "prevent absorption of unwanted sugar"; (13) *Thyro-Vital*, claimed to "improve thyroid function"; (14) Jerusalem Artichoke Capsules, an Edgar Cayce product described as "a natural equivalent to insulin injections"; and (15) *Mummy Food* (nuggets consisting of figs, dates, and cornmeal). The "Better Nutrition" section of the Home Health Products, Inc., Winter 1992 catalog states:

> Mummy Food has a fascinating history. In a dream that Edgar Cayce had concerning the discovery of ancient records in Egypt, a mummy came to life to help him translate these records. This mummy gave directions for the preparation of food that she required, thus the name "mummy food.". . . For particular individuals [Cayce] stated that it was "almost a spiritual food."

The company's brochure states: "In addition to changes in diet, Edgar Cayce frequently recommended specific remedies and treatments. Many of these had to be custom-formulated from herbs, oils, and other naturally occurring substances."

The A.R.E. Bookstore, which sells direct and by mail, features many books by or about Cayce, including the twenty-four-volume "library series" of excerpts from his readings, usually priced at $395. It also carries a large selection of books and tapes on psychic and metaphysical topics, including dream interpretation, reincarnation, tarot, *I Ching,* and pyramid power.

Another item sold by the bookstore is the *Physician's Reference Notebook*, by William A. McGarey, M.D., and associates. In its third printing in 1988, the book offers treatment recommendations based on the Cayce readings for over fifty diseases and conditions, including baldness, breast cancer, color blindness, diabetes, hemophilia, hydrocephalus, leukemia, multiple sclerosis, muscular dystrophy, stroke, stuttering, and syphilis. An A.R.E. mailing to chiropractors during the 1980s stated:

> This book is a "magic tool" to be used in conjunction with your professional skill and knowledge in healing some of your more difficult cases. One of our colleagues, using the information in our commentaries, has cured dozens of psoriasis cases. . . . Even some of the neurological degenerative conditions, such as M.S. [multiple sclerosis], A.L.S. [amyotrophic lateral sclerosis], or even . . . [foot drop] have responded exceptionally well to these recommendations.

According to the *Notebook*: (1) baldness is most often caused by glandular insufficiency and spinal lesions (subluxations); (2) color blindness is caused by the conduct of the afflicted person in a past life, and treatment should include spinal adjustments and a diet consisting mostly of alkali-producing foods; (3) hemophilia is correctable, "a simple case of a deep-seated defect in the assimilations of the body," and treatment of newborns so afflicted should consist primarily in the addition of blood pudding to the diet; (4) obesity is caused principally by an excess of starches in the diet, and treatment should include the elimination of most starches; and (5) psoriasis is caused by a thinning of the intestinal walls, which "allows toxic products from the intestinal tract to leak into the circulatory system and find their way into the lymph flow of the skin."

Channels of the "Great Healer"?

In 1970, William A. McGarey, M.D., and his wife, Gladys McGarey, M.D., founded the nonprofit A.R.E. Clinic in Phoenix, Arizona. According to an article in *Medical World News*, they opened the facility to offer "comprehensive care to patients seeking holistic medical alternatives." Later, Gladys McGarey resigned as clinic co-director and set up another "holistic" practice in Scottsdale, Arizona, with their physician-daughter.

A founding member of the American Holistic Medical Association, William McGarey is currently board chairman of the clinic. In an interview in *Health Talks* (1989), he said that the clinic had a staff of forty-five or fifty persons, including five physicians (one an osteopath), a chiropractor, and a psychologist with a doctoral degree. An advertisement for the clinic in the January/February 1992 issue of *East West Natural Health* names two naturopaths.

In the *Health Talks* interview, McGarey denied any conflict or contradiction between his Cayce-based practices and his medical education. "The philosophy behind the A.R.E. clinic," he said, "is that everyone is a whole human being . . . created in the image of God." According to McGarey, the clinic consists of a general practice; a "brain injury center" (that is, a "Neurological Improvement Program" for individuals who suffer from, for example, cerebral palsy or autism); and an "energy medicine center that looks at the biomagnetic energies of the body." The clinic offers, in part, "electromagnetic field therapy," relaxation training, the laying on of hands, and the residential Temple Beautiful Program. McGarey described this as an eleven-day "rejuvenation program" that includes dream analysis, stress reduction, visualization, biofeedback, exercise, nutrition, and supplementation. A 1991 brochure stated that the program had been conducted more than two hundred times over the past decade and accommodates ten to fifteen participants. It costs $4,100. In 1990, the clinic began offering Physician Telephone Consultations, which cost $50 per session of fifteen to sixty minutes.

In *Health Talks* McGarey lamented: "When doctors fail to recognize the spiritual aspect of the human being, they miss the most important part." When one recognizes our destiny as "getting back to our spiritual origin," he said, "there is a different kind of emphasis on healing; you do not get tied up with modalities. Healing is more of a spiritual event." McGarey also stated that when treating someone, "we cannot consider ourselves as the healer. We are only the . . . channel of the Great Healer."

"Most any kind of condition," he declared, "is not as significant as the cause and what we can do to direct the body back to normal." He further stated that "any time you are disturbing what is normal, you are creating disease" (an orientation apparently shared by Natural Hygiene). In *Edgar Cayce Remedies* (1983), McGarey advocates application of potato poultices to the eyes for cataracts, monthly "high-colonic" enemas for angina pectoris, and castor oil packs for epilepsy and cat bites. In his column in the November/December 1991 *Venture Inward*, he proclaims: "There is no death, and true health is found in the consciousness of the Oneness we have with that Creative Source."

The Cayce Way to "Wellness"

Each year, A.R.E. holds dozens of conferences in Virginia Beach and various other cities. They have covered such subjects as angels, astrology ("the key to self-discovery"), chakra healing, "intuitive healing," reincarnation, UFOs, weight control, and "holistic" financial management. A flyer for a 1992 "psychic training" seminar states: "You are already psychic. . . .You only need to become aware of it!" According to a form letter I received from A.R.E. in 1991, half of those who attend these conferences are newcomers.

On September 8, 1990, I attended an A.R.E. "Special Event" entitled "Wellness: The Cayce Approach to Health and Healing," held in the cafeteria of the Baptist-denomination Riverside Church in Manhattan, near Columbia University. "Tuition" at the door was $89. I estimated that three hundred people were present, most of them white and apparently over the age of thirty. Books for sale covered two tables near the cafeteria entrance. I was accompanied by a social worker from India with a master's degree in theology, who likened the atmosphere to that of a Christian retreat.

Opening remarks were made by Charles Thomas Cayce, who said the Edgar Cayce tradition is at the midpoint on a continuum where Christian Science and conventional medicine lie at either extreme. He asked us to rate the applicability of twenty-five items on a "health inventory" included in a scanty information packet. The items include: (1) "I have a sense of well-being"; (2) "I do not depend on medicines, including prescription drugs, to maintain my health"; (3) "Silence is enjoyable"; and (4) "I have a personal definition of God which has meaning to me." Then he told us to take a few minutes to discuss one negative response with someone nearby.

Dr. Cayce said the conference would take "a closer look at alternative explanations for illness [and] alternative approaches to wellness." He stated that over two thirds of the readings given by his grandfather concerned illnesses and their cure, and that another large portion dealt with general health considerations, such as "emotional imbalance" and "attunement of the body and the mind to the spiritual aspect of ourselves."

He explained that in the Cayce readings, the word "spirit" is used interchangeably with the terms "God," "creative forces," and "life force," and that this force can be used in "good ways or bad ways that we label evil." He then spoke of the "universal Christ-consciousness," which he defined as "an awareness within each soul imprinting its pattern on the mind, waiting to be awakened by the will, of our oneness with God."

"The premise here," he explained "is that the mind is more than brain, cortex, blood, cells." He defined healing as "the process of awakening the God-pattern within," and recited a phrase common in the Cayce readings: "Spirit is the life, mind is the builder, the physical is the result." He said that with every thought we have, we are building patterns—"thought forms"— that "create a mental body, an energy body . . . a nonphysical body manifesting as colors and images" perceptible to "people with various sorts of sensitivities."

The next speaker was Eric Mein, M.D., a former "Fellow-in-Residence" at the Edgar Cayce Foundation, who was finishing his medical residency at the University of Washington in Seattle. Mein led us in breathing and stretching exercises while the slide projector and screen were being readied. Then he wondered aloud why it is "unheard-of" for the "spirit-body connection" to be discussed in conventional medical circles. He referred to the temples of Asclepius, the Greek god of healing, which were numerous in the ancient world, as "holistic centers." Mein suggested that everything affects the immune system but then dismissed the details of a pivotal diagrammatic slide as "gibberish."

Gladys McGarey was next. In addition to having co-founded the A.R.E. Clinic, she has also been president of the American Holistic Medical Association. Her topic was "The Healing Energy of Pain." After characterizing her dog as "a real pain" but still her friend, she declared that pain itself was indeed "our friend"—because, she explained, it awakens within us "the awareness that we're alive. If you don't feel pain . . . you're dead." Her conception of pain, she said, comprises not only physical pain, but "mental pain," such as the pain of confusion, "the pain of forgetting" (as in Alzheimer's disease), and the "pain that comes from remembering."

McGarey recounted the story of a mother whose infant had been hospitalized and near death from a large cyst on her right lung. "It didn't look like the baby was going to make it through the night. We called our study group and had the . . . group begin to pray for [them]." The mother "got up to go to the hospital, but as she walked past her bed, she laid on the bed and she fell asleep. About half an hour later she woke up just throwing up this huge amount of mucus . . . but again she fell back asleep and she didn't wake up until morning." Then she called the hospital and was told that her baby was "doing much better." The next morning an x-ray revealed that the baby's lung was clear. "You see," McGarey explained, "what had happened was that the mother took on her baby's condition and she threw up a lot of mucus that cleared the situation for the baby."

Of another patient, who had had "severe" lung cancer and had been very angry and miserable, she said: "It was his anger, actually, that had probably precipitated his cancer." Although he had died within two months of the diagnosis, McGarey judged that massage and other "alternative" therapies had been successful because the patient had died "in a completely connected state." She also expressed belief in reincarnation, "past-life regression," and "the chakra system," which she equated with the endocrine system.

Mein and McGarey were joined by Roger Jahnke, C.A., O.M.D., for a panel discussion and question-and-answer session moderated by Cayce. The initials after Jahnke's name stand for "Certified Acupuncturist" and "Doctor of Oriental Medicine." Then a teacher at the unaccredited Santa Barbara College of Oriental Medicine, he said that as a premed student he had worked in various hospital departments, including dietary, but had never found what "true healing was all about." So he "dropped out basically," became an English major, and started writing poetry. In the literature of aboriginal cultures, he had found that "the spiritual tradition and the medicine are one." In response to a question, Mein stated that chronic fatigue syndrome is often the result of "impaired eliminations" or "toxic buildup" and suggested a diet limited to a single food, such as apples. Jahnke recommended tai chi, a Chinese martial art comprising ballet-like exercises. Near the discussion's end, Cayce asked the panelists whether they considered "past-life influences" in the process of diagnosing their patients. Mein replied "sometimes," and McGarey said yes.

"All the Good Stuff, Medicare Doesn't Pay For"

After lunch, Jahnke instructed us in acupressure, "personal reflexology," and "freestyle" tai chi. "After you get into this . . . new health care revolution," he said, "if you get confused about what to do . . . go to the Chinese literature, or go to the Ayurvedic Hindu-Buddhist literature, or go to the Native American literature, or go to the Polynesian literature. Go to any . . . health literature of any [aboriginal] culture." Jahnke emphasized that his "self-applied health-enhancement methods" could be learned in

just a few minutes and "can't be forgotten because [they] are so deep within
. . . your cellular nature." But in fact it took him about forty-five minutes
to teach the methods only superficially—and quite forgettably.

"We've paid too much for health care," he lamented. "Somebody was
complaining earlier: 'All the good stuff, Medicare doesn't pay for.'" After
teaching "alternate nostril breathing," he marveled aloud that Edgar
Cayce—who had traveled very little—had known about the practice: "It
just was one of the first things that blew my mind. I mean, there he was in
Hopkinsville, Kentucky, and maybe the circus came to town, and maybe
there was a Buddhist monk in the side show—but maybe not."

A woman in the audience inquired about the significance of "very
extra-long ear lobes." Jahnke replied that if she had such ear lobes, she
"may be a relative of the Buddha." In response to the laughter, he assured
us he wasn't joking. With regard to herbal tonics, he stated: "Be sure you
know what you're taking—and then go ahead because the herbs are good."
Although "we love all this esoteric stuff," he said, the salient message of
the day is that healing takes an investment of time and that we should not
interfere with healing by taking too many medicines.

Later, Jahnke told us to pinch our fingers to discover tenderness at
acupuncture points. A woman reported some in her pinky, which Jahnke
said was the channel for the heart and the small intestine. He advised her
to "eat good," love herself, and "get a little exercise." He informed us that
acupuncture points lie throughout the palm of the hand and told us to "find
a sore spot." My companion apparently tried too hard and noted his palm
was "sore all over."

A question from the audience prompted Jahnke's return to the subject
of herbs, which he described as "super-nutrients because our food is kind
of in trouble," even in health-food stores. Vitamin supplements, however,
"are a little difficult" because they are extracted from their source. "In
herbal medicine," he said, "you're deriving the full nutritional benefit,
especially if the herbs are concentrated in a very special way." But he was
evasive when asked to give an example of a tonic herb, calling the question
"inappropriate" and repeating his earlier recommendation that interested
persons sign a sheet at the information table.

During the last break, an anxious-looking woman hurriedly handed
me a business card advertising a Reverend Jean's channeling classes.

The final presentation described the Cayce home remedies, a collection of sixteen methods detailed in a videotape covered by the cost of
admission. They include: (1) castor oil packs, "to help with arthritis, colds,
gallstones, ulcers, and more"; (2) peanut oil massages, "to prevent arthri-

tis"; (3) potato poultices, "to relieve tired or strained eyes"; (4) castor oil liniments, "to remove warts"; and (5) coffee-ground foot baths, "to soothe sore feet and improve circulation in the legs."

Way "Beyond Medicine"

Parapsychology popularizer Hans Holzer, Ph.D., has called Cayce the "greatest of all dietetic healers." In *Beyond Medicine* (1987), he writes: "Edgar Cayce abundantly made clear in his writings [that] certain combinations of foodstuffs are chemically incompatible in the human system [and] can create damage or at the very least ill health." Holzer gives two examples of such incompatibility according to Cayce: (1) coffee should be taken black or with hot milk, but not with cold milk; and (2) tea with sugar, especially white sugar, is hepatotoxic, while tea with honey is not.

According to an A.R.E. Clinic chart:

- 80 percent of one's daily food intake should consist of: fruits and fruit juices, vegetables, water, and herbal teas;

- 20 percent should consist of dairy products (including whole milk and butter), whole-grain breads, high-fiber cereals (including granola), honey, soups. fowl, lamb, and fish;

- one serving about three times per week should suffice for beef, brown rice, oils, potatoes with skin, cheese, eggs, spices, gelatin products, and desserts (e.g., ice cream); and

- fried foods, alcohol, pasta, white bread, pork, and "processed foods" should be avoided—except "crisp bacon," which may be eaten occasionally.

The excerpts from "readings" in *Edgar Cayce on Diet and Health* include the following tidbits:

- Canned tomatoes are usually preferable to fresh.

- Gelatin enhances glandular activity.

- Certified raw milk is to be preferred, unless it came from cows that eat certain types of weeds or grass growing in January.

- Raw green peppers should not be eaten without other foods.

- One's diet should consist of 80 percent alkaline-producing and 20 percent acid-producing foods.

- Citrus fruits and cereals should not be eaten together.

- No combination whatsoever of white bread, potatoes, and spaghetti should be eaten at the same meal.

- Ice cream is far preferable to pie, which combines starches and sweets.

- Orange juice and milk should be drunk separately at opposite ends of the day.

- It is better to consume meats with sweets than with starches.

- Neither citrus juices nor tomato juice should be consumed with any starch other than whole-wheat bread.

- Ideally, lime juice should be added to orange juice, and lemon juice to grapefruit juice (an idea, the authors admitted, "probably new to those working in the science of modern dietetics and food research").

- It is "normal" to consume above-ground and below-ground vegetables in a ratio of three to one.

- Squirrel should be stewed or well cooked.

- Cheese and cream are "good for the system."

- Beet and "raw" cane sugars are the best.

The book's foreword stresses that all the readings it contains pertain to "normal," healthy people who are not overweight.

Another book published the same year, *Edgar Cayce Speaks*, is a cross-referenced encyclopedia of excerpts from Cayce readings pertaining to foods and beverages. In the foreword, William McGarey says that Cayce's physiological notions are "strange concepts." Cayce recommended consumption of yogurt to "purify" the alimentary canal, saying it would add "vital forces." He also stated that Jerusalem artichoke (a tuber), if taken once every ten days, would eradicate the tendency toward dark circles under the eyes. However, two caveats are spelled out by Cayce himself: First, "That which might be applicable to [one person] should not . . . even be considered for others; unless their own condition is in that state of being parallel with this [person]." (The editor adds: "the determination that a state of being is 'parallel' is a complex and subtle problem and ought not to be made lightly.") Second, "It isn't so much *what* the body eats as it is the *combinations* that are taken at times. Beware then of those things."

"Sounds Like Hogwash"

In *Health and Healing: Understanding Conventional and Alternative Medicine* (1983), ethnopharmacologist Andrew Weil, M.D., a staunch "natural medicine" proponent, says of the Cayce readings:

> Much of this material sounds like hogwash. I, for one, do not expect California to fall into the sea by 1998, creating a new coast near Phoenix, Arizona. I find many of Cayce's metabolic and hormonal explanations of specific diseases to be garbled and fanciful, such as his assertion that multiple sclerosis is an imbalance of the endocrine glands due to deficiency of gold.

The Bottom Line

The effect on our society of nonsense as diverse, intricate, and profuse as that of the Edgar Cayce tradition is incalculable. As far as I know, however, no study has been conducted to determine the extent to which Cayce advocates follow his advice or what impact their practices have on their lives. Nor has it been determined whether they seek appropriate medical intervention when it is needed. The A.R.E. dietary philosophy, derived from the readings—which in turn were supposedly derived from the "collective consciousness" or whatnot—is nebulous, internally contradictory, and possibly conducive to chronic confusion.

6

The Ayurvedic
Medicine Men

"Americans Turn to Maharishi Ayur-Veda"

This is the title of the lead article in the February/March 1992 issue of *To Your Health*, a newsletter distributed free by Maharishi Ayur-Veda Products International, Inc. (MAPI), in Lancaster, Massachusetts. According to the article, "Maharishi Ayur-Veda differs from other holistic systems." It is supposedly "the traditional knowledge of Ayur-Veda, the timeless science of life, which has been restored to its original purity and completeness by Maharishi Mahesh Yogi, the founder of the Transcendental Meditation program, working with the world's foremost Ayurvedic physicians." One goal of Maharishi Ayur-Veda—"to achieve world peace by creating peace on the level of the individual"—is similar to that of macrobiotics.

Will the Real Allopathy Please Stand Up?

Webster's New Collegiate Dictionary defines allopathy as "a system of medical practice making use of all measures proved of value in the treatment of disease"—in other words, scientific medicine. But the term was coined by vitalist and empiricist Samuel Christian Hahnemann (1755-1843) to disparage conventional medicine and distinguish it from his own school of practice, which he called homeopathy. One of homeopathy's premises, Hahnemann's "Law of Similars," holds that "like cures like." At

79

the turn of the eighteenth century, Hahnemann propagated his belief that tiny amounts of substances that can cause symptoms in healthy people can cure the diseases that have these symptoms. This conclusion was based largely on the results of self-experimentation that followed his observation that quinine—which can produce thirst, fever, and throbbing headache—can cure malaria, which has similar symptoms.

The Greek-derived prefix *allo* means "other" or "different"; *pathy* means "disease." Hahnemann described the orthodox medical tradition of his time as allopathic because he perceived no consistent or logical relationship between the conventional drugs prescribed and the symptoms in question. He also used the term "antipathy" to denote "treatment by contraries," or the doctrine of opposites, which may be thought of as an allopathic subcategory.

While the earliest writings on food and food-related practices come from ancient Egypt, the oldest documents that describe human nutrition and dietetics originated in India with Ayurvedic medicine. Although it encompasses a form of homeopathy, Ayurvedic medicine is better categorized as allopathic because it mainly involves modalities thought to produce effects different from symptoms. *Ayur* derives from the Sanskrit *ayus*, meaning "life" or "life span"; *veda* has been interpreted as "knowledge," "science," and "sacred lore." Thus, Ayurveda is supposedly the science of life or longevity.

Ayurvedic medicine is rooted in four Sanskrit books called the Vedas, which are the oldest and most important scriptures of India. The Vedas were shaped prior to 500 B.C.E. by tribes of Sanskrit-speaking people who had invaded India about a thousand years earlier. These were the Aryans (literally, "noble ones"), who, incidentally, consumed beef and alcoholic beverages. The Vedas were thought to have been revealed by the godhead (Brahma) to Aryan sages, who passed them on by word of mouth. They consist of hymns and chants, prayers and curses, incantations, and magico-religious poems. The oldest and most sacred of the Vedas, the *Rg-veda* (also called the *Rig* or *Rik Veda),* was composed between 1500 and 900 B.C. E. and includes more than a thousand hymns. Most of these are addressed to various gods (especially the war-god Indra), but one is addressed to frogs. The hymns were intended for recitation during animal sacrifices, at which a hallucinogenic beverage was drunk. According to A.L. Basham, the late Oriental studies scholar, the phrasing of the hymns is not significant: "It is the holy sound that counts."

In *Mythology's Last Gods* (1992), William Harwood states that the light-skinned, priestly conquerers of India, the Brahmana, promoted the

Vedas to prevent rebellion in the lower castes. He further writes that the Vedas "decreed death or torture for even the mildest attempt to claim equality with a member of a higher caste, but offered the certainty of eventual reincarnation as a Brahmana to unquestioning Uncle Toms."

Vedic medicine developed as a combination of religious, magical, and empirical views and practices. The causes of disease include sin, violation of a norm, the unjust cursing of a fellow man, and the wrongs committed by one's parents or by "oneself" in a previous incarnation. Disease is either punishment meted out by the gods directly or through demons, or the result of witchcraft. Remedies include prayer, sacrifice, magic, exorcism, and water as a "purifier." Numerous diseases are mentioned in the Vedas, but they are not described in detail. According to the Vedas, the world is not matter but spirit, moral perfection is the only means of salvation, and sickness denotes individual culpability.

The religious-dietary *Dharma-Sutra* texts proscribe consumption of many foods, including:

- all foods offered or given by an actor, hypocrite, musician, physician, police officer, woman without a male relative, anyone accused of a mortal sin, and other assorted persons;

- all foods specifically prepared for another person;

- all foods smelled by a cow;

- all meat from animals that are tame or wander alone;

- garlic, leek, onion, turnip, duck, and many other miscellaneous items.

The Beatles' "Simple" Mistake

The title "Maharishi" combines two Sanskrit words meaning "great seer (clairvoyant or prophet)." Ayurvedic medicine's chief patron, the Maharishi Mahesh Yogi, was born in 1911 in Uttar Kashi, India. His world headquarters is in the Netherlands. After attending Allahabad University in India, he became a monk and for thirteen years studied mysticism in the Himalayas. After his guru's death in 1953, he retreated to a cave, where he lived for two years.

The Maharishi's "Spiritual Regeneration" movement, which was renamed the Transcendental Meditation movement, began in India in 1955. According to *TM: Discovering Inner Energy and Overcoming Stress* (1975), by Harold H. Bloomfield, M.D., and associates, in 1958 the

Maharishi "proclaimed the possibility of all humanity's attaining enlightenment" and inaugurated a "World Plan" intended to encompass "every individual on earth." Shortly thereafter, he embarked upon a world tour to spread his teachings.

The spread of Hindu thought to the West escalated in the 1960s and 1970s. In the 1960s, the Maharishi taught the Beatles how to meditate. Later in that decade, a group of students practicing his brand of meditation inveigled their way into an experiment conducted by a prestigious Harvard researcher, who concluded that TM could be used to lower blood pressure. Basically, the practice of TM involves sitting in a comfortable position with one's eyes closed for fifteen to twenty minutes twice a day. The meditator mentally repeats a "mantra" supposedly chosen expressly for him or her by the teacher. Mantras are "secret" words representing Hindu deities and believed to possess magical power.

In *The Lives of John Lennon* (1988), Albert Goldman states that the Beatles became converts of the Maharishi in 1967, after attending a lecture in London in which he had alleged that TM could effect rejuvenescence. The following day, with the Rolling Stones' Mick Jagger and pop singer Marianne Faithful, they accompanied the "holy one" on a railroad trip to Wales to take a five-day course in TM. There the Beatles came to the Maharishi's defense against the derisive questions of a hostile press and publicly renounced drugs in favor of TM. "Maharishi" soon became a household word.

In February 1968, the Beatles flew from England to India to join their new guru at his Meditation Academy. Goldman writes: "Here they found not the primitive shelter of twigs and leaves prescribed by Hindu tradition or the free tuition that is the duty of the holy man to provide but instead a $350-a-day Western-style resort hotel, where each Beatle was assigned a chalet with hot and cold running water, four-poster bed, and electric heaters." Ringo Starr described the center as very luxurious. With the Beatles were many rich, elderly Swedish women, some "pretty girls" from California, folk singer Donovan Leitch, the Beach Boys' Mike Love, and actress Mia Farrow, then newly divorced. Goldman concludes that the press treated the goings-on at the academy as hokum and strove to present the Maharishi as dishonest.

According to Goldman, the Maharishi would deposit donations from his disciples into a Swiss bank account under his own name. Goldman writes:

> Once he had hooked the Beatles, the guru began to speak of a worldwide network of meditation centers that could accommodate

millions of people. When pressed about his business ambitions, the wily guru would explain that he had to be active now because soon he would "retire into silence."

The Beatles wrote virtually all the songs for their so-called "White Album" within two months at the academy. But Paul McCartney left displaying a lack of commitment, and the remaining Beatles became disillusioned when they discovered that the Maharishi had seduced one of the young Californians staying at the academy. They departed the day after their discovery. Upon his return to England, John Lennon announced: "We made a mistake. What could be more simple?" Yet more than twenty years later, in 1992, both George Harrison and Ringo Starr performed at a British concert promoting the Maharishi's Natural Law Party.

The Fourth Phase

Through the 1970s, the leading "New Age" theoreticians—including Swami Rama, another major supporter of Ayurvedic medicine—appeared one after another. Not to be outdone, the Maharishi claimed he could teach advanced meditators to levitate. In the Spring 1989 *Skeptical Inquirer*, Indian magician B. Premanand reports that in 1977 he challenged the Maharishi to fly by his own power over a distance of about two miles. The Maharishi said he would do so if paid the equivalent of about $1,000, which he believed Premanand and his skeptics group could not afford. However, when they returned the next day with the money, the Maharishi declined to take flight, declaring that TM is not for demonstration purposes. According to the National Council Against Health Fraud's March/April 1991 newsletter, "Paraplegics have been bilked by promises that with enough TM training they would eventually rise from their wheelchairs by levitation." Other alleged benefits of TM and TM-Sidhi (advanced TM) have included elephantine strength, perfect health, immortality, "mastery over nature," "naturally correct" social behavior, and the powers of invisibility, immateriality, and telepathy.

In 1977, sociologist Eric Woodrum identified three phases of the TM movement in the United States. From 1959 to 1965, TM was interpreted as the central component in a program of spiritual development leading to nirvana—complete detachment from the material world, attainable only via the extinction of individuality. The program included yoga, silent prayer, dietary practices, and attendance at meditation courses. During the next four years the movement expanded rapidly as it won major publicity by linking with aspects of the counterculture. The goal of "cosmic consciousness" was redefined as bliss, energy, and peace, without reference to material nonattachment. Since 1970, the movement has downplayed otherworldliness (at public introductory levels) and emphasized practical, physiological, material, and social benefits of TM for conventional people. It produces a steady flow of "scientific validation" through an organizational arm, Maharishi International University. TM is also promoted through the American Foundation for the Science of Creative Intelligence, the World Plan Executive Council, and the World Medical Association for Perfect Health. Maharishi Ayur-Veda seems to have been born in 1980.

"Happy Thoughts . . . Happy Molecules"

In 1985, the Maharishi began marketing a variety of products and services under the trademark "Maharishi Ayur-Veda," which now include *Maharishi Amrit Kalash* ("the perfect nutritional food"), herbal teas and seasonings based on Ayurvedic body types, candy, beauty aids, "aromatherapy" oils, Vedic music cassettes, videotapes, and incense—all obtainable via a 24-hour toll-free order line. The Maharishi has also announced plans for immense theme parks called "Veda Land" in Canada, Brazil, India, Japan and Florida (next to Disney World), but none of these has materialized.

The information packet I received from MAPI in 1991 included an audiocassette titled "On Creating Health: An Introduction to Maharishi Ayur-Veda." It features an interview with Ayurvedic superstar Deepak Chopra, M.D. Conducted by National Football League Hall-of-Famer Joe Namath, the interview is interspersed with both narration and comments made by unidentified persons lauding Ayurveda.

"According to Maharishi Ayur-Veda," said Chopra, "it is consciousness which conceives, constructs, and actually becomes the physical body .... Our thoughts are really processes that become molecules. If you have happy thoughts, then you make happy molecules. On the other hand, if you have sad thoughts and angry thoughts and hostile thoughts, then you make those molecules, which may depress the immune system, and make you more susceptible to disease."

The narrator describes Maharishi Ayur-Veda as "the modern rediscovery of this ancient system of natural medicine. Ayurveda was at the root of much of ancient Greek medicine, which in turn is the root of modern medicine. Ayurveda locates the infinite intelligence of nature, which structures the entire universe in human consciousness, and uses this knowledge to bring life into accord with natural law. Ayurveda also finds the intelligence of nature in the plant kingdom, and restores perfect balance to the body through proper nutrition, along with special therapies and herbal preparations." Later, the narrator states:

> Maharishi Ayur-Veda brings to modern medical care a time-tested and complete knowledge of prevention and treatment of disease, the preservation of health, and the promotion of longevity. . . . The treatments are natural, free of harmful side effects, and truly holistic. Ayur-Veda eliminates disease at its source, rather than working at the superficial level of symptoms.

On the reverse side of the tape, the Maharishi himself speaks: "All systems in the world will find Ayur-Veda a great friend, a great nourishing feature for life to be enjoyed in perfect health, and the world to be enjoyed in perfect peace and harmony in the family of nations."

In January 1993, *To Your Health* announced that that the term "Ayur-Veda" in MAPI's name and logo had been changed to "Ayur-Ved."

At the Maharishi's Request

Endocrinologist Deepak Chopra, M.D., arrived on the Ayur-Veda scene in 1985. In that year, according to an article in the May/June 1990 *In Health*, he met the Maharishi, who persuaded him to found the American Association of Ayurvedic Medicine and become medical director of the Maharishi Ayur-Veda Health Center for Behavioral Medicine and Stress Management in Lancaster, Massachusetts. Chopra's quest, the *In Health* article states, is "to restore modern medicine's soul"; and his approach is to "heal the psyche," since the body "can heal itself." Chopra calls himself the "chief messenger" of Ayurvedic medicine, and it is no wonder that he is, what with the Maharishi's public relations machine behind him. He describes his Ayurvedic approach as "mysticism with a scientific watchdog."

In *New Techniques of Inner Healing* (1992), a collection of interviews with "masters of alternative healing," Chopra stated: "We are thoughts that have learned how to create the physical machine, the body." In an interview for *Better World* published in 1992, Chopra declared: "There is no physical world. It's all projection. The whole thing is a Quantum Soup."

Chopra's books include *Creating Health* (1987), *Return of the Rishi* (1988), *Quantum Healing* (1989), *Perfect Health: The Complete Mind/ Body Guide* (1990), and *Unconditional Life: Mastering the Forces that*

Shape Personal Reality (1991). All except the last are dedicated to his guru, the Maharishi. (When I phoned Chopra's office in September 1992 to inquire about this inconsistency, a representative told me that although the book is indeed not dedicated to the Maharishi, no inconsistency exists. In any case, the book affirmatively cites and quotes the Maharishi.) The following statements are excerpted from *Creating Health.*

- The old [scientific] model of the body . . . must be discarded, because that model keeps us in the grips of disease, aging, and ignorance. . . . Knowledge [of the "mind-body connection"] is too huge to be straitjacketed by medical science.

- Food transformed, given consciousness, is us.

- The intelligence of our bodies knows what [food] is good for it.

- Reality exists because you agree to it.

In the second edition of *Creating Health* (1991), Chopra describes the "hundredth monkey phenomenon" to support his belief in a "collective consciousness." Named after a folk tale, the "hundredth monkey" story was reported by "New Age" author Lyall Watson in his book, *Lifetide* (1979), and was popularized by human-potential guru Ken Keyes, Jr., in *The Hundredth Monkey* (1982). It concerns monkeys on a Japanese island who were given sweet potatoes by researchers. One of them began to wash the grit off the potatoes, others gradually followed suit, and when a "critical mass" was reached, nearly all the rest suddenly adopted the practice—and so did monkeys on other islands. Paranormalists consider the story evidence of "group consciousness," but science philosopher Ron Amundson inspected the detailed records of direct observers and concluded that Watson had greatly exaggerated what had taken place.

In *Perfect Health,* Chopra writes that attainment of perfect health "is only a question of following the silent river of intelligence to its source." He advocates TM, aromatherapy, and "purification" programs. Early in 1991, it was reported that *Perfect Health* had sold 80,000 copies and was in its sixth printing, and that the Maharishi Ayur-Veda Health Center in Lancaster, Massachusetts, was booked up to a year in advance. Thirteen similar centers in the United States had had more than 100,000 clients in the six years since they had begun opening. A profile of Chopra in the January/February 1992 *American Health* states that twelve to fourteen new patients per week undergo diagnosis and treatment at the Massachusetts center, at a cost of $2,500 to $4,300 or more per person.

Sense of "Humors"

Ayurvedic theory and practice are complex, but the principal Ayurvedic theory—that of *tridosha*—regards the human body as composed of five "elements": earth, air, fire, water, and ether. The preponderance of these elements determines various constitutional types, each prone to ailments due to a deficiency or excess of one or more elements. The fundamental constitutional types are *pitta*, *kapha*, and *vata*. These terms also designate the fundamental physiological forces—"humors" (body fluids) or *doshas*— postulated to characterize the types. *Pitta*—"fire" or "bile"—said to be a combination of fire and water, is analogous to yang. *Kapha*—"mucus," "phlegm," or "water humor"—said to be a combination of earth and water, is analogous to yin. *Vata* (or *vayu*)—"wind" or "air humor"—said to be a combination of air and "space," is believed to mediate between *pitta* and *kapha*. The *doshas* were identified with the three supposed universal forces: sun, moon, and wind.

The symptoms of excessive *pitta* are said to include anemia, ca-chexia, diarrhea, fainting, fever, indigestion, nausea, vomiting, and gener-alized weakness. Insufficiency of *pitta* results in slowed digestion. Exces-sive *kapha* supposedly can cause anorexia, asthma, bronchitis, drowsiness, emaciation, fever, and vomiting, while excessive *vata* can cause anorexia, diarrhea, fever, and generalized weakness. Fever and weakness thus are common to all excesses.

Treatment purportedly balances these three forces *(doshas)* through meditation, diet, botanicals, specific exercises, and other means. Accord-ing to Ayurveda, *prana*, the "life force," is obtained from both food and the atmosphere. The Ayurvedic diet consists mainly of grains, ghee (a semi-fluid clarified butter), and certain vegetables. One principle of Ayurvedic nutrition is that food should be heated or cooked and consumed while it is hot.

Ayurvedic nutrition is concerned basically with "constitutional type," specific food characteristics, and the season of the year. Significant food characteristics include "taste" (sweet, sour, salty, pungent, bitter, or astringent), temperature, oiliness/dryness, and liquidity/solidity. By Ayur-vedic standards, foods believed capable of intensifying a particular dosha should not be consumed during the season in which the dosha predomi-nates: Consumption of spicy, pungent foods in summer is thought to intensify *pitta*; dry fruits and high-protein foods in autumn, *vata*; and cold drinks and dairy products in winter, *kapha*. For excess of *pitta*, astringent, bitter, and sweet foods are prescribed—e.g., beans, wheat and other grains, sweet milk, and bitter herbs. For excess of *kapha*, astringent, bitter, and pungent foods are prescribed—e.g., beans (again), hot spices, and acidic fruits. For excess of *vata*, acidic, salty, and sweet foods are prescribed— e.g., wheat (again), milk (again), acidic fruits (again), warm drinks, and sweet vegetables.

Ayurvedic medicine and mysticism appear inseparable no matter who the guru is. In the July 17, 1992 issue of *News India*, D.K.M. Kartha presents fifteen "wisdom sayings" specifically related to food and nutrition. These include:

- "Exercise and moderate, nutritious food—these two are earthly incarnations of the twin gods of health in heaven, the Aswini Devas. I follow these two and do not, therefore, depend on doctors."

- "There is no medicine that is as potent as proper food. It is possible to cure illness simply through correct nutrition."

In *Diet and Nutrition: A Holistic Approach* (1978), Rudolph Ballentine, M.D., writes:

Eating raw food in the quantities that were necessary to sustain his high degree of physical activity, primitive man was probably required to eat frequently. In fact, according to some writers, he ate almost constantly. . . . As a result, his consciousness was more continuously focused on the intake of food and its digestion. As man became more civilized, he invested more of his consciousness in higher pursuits. He came to understand that the cooking fire helped him with his digestion and also permitted the concentration of food into a few discrete feedings through the day so that the rest of the time he need not be occupied with matters of food.

He also states:

From the ancient Eastern perspective, consciousness is potentially much more capable of influencing the way the body functions and the way it handles food than is the food itself. . . . The Eastern point of view relegates diet to an inferior place in the scheme of variables affecting the human being.

Preventive Medicine?

As for the "other means" of balancing the three doshas: Traditionally, when diet therapy proved inefficacious, or when the illness was severe, fasting, emetics, "drastic" purgatives, and bloodletting were brought to bear against the disease. Indeed, they were considered preventive medicine: an emetic biweekly, a purgative every month, and bloodletting twice a year. In traditional Ayurveda, alcoholism, anorexia, nausea, indigestion, ascites, and edema are treated with goat feces washed with urine; constipation is treated with a mixture of milk and urine; impotence is treated with 216 kinds of enemas (some including the testicles of peacocks, swans, and turtles); and epilepsy and insanity are treated with ass urine.

For health maintenance, proponents of Maharishi Ayur-Veda recommend training courses in TM and TM-Sidhi for a total cost of $3,400, instruction in the Maharishi Psychophysiological and Primordial Sound Techniques for $1,400, and three weeks of *panchakarma* annually for $2,700 to $6,600. In *Perfect Health*, Chopra defines *panchakarma* as "purification treatment," the goal of which is to rid the body of *ama* ("residual impurities deposited in the cells as the result of improper digestion"). Chopra further defines *mental ama* as "impure or negative thoughts or moods" and lists six steps of panchakarma: (1) "oleation," the ingestion of clarified butter or a medicated oil "to soften up the doshas and minimize digestive action"; (2) administration of a laxative to reduce *pitta*; (3) oil massage, the oil "herbalized" according to constitutional type; (4) "herbalized" steam treatments; (5) administration of medicated enemas (Ayurveda "lists well over a hundred") to "flush the loosened doshas out through the intestinal tract"; and (6) inhalation of medicinal oils or herbal mixtures. In *Prakruti: Your Ayurvedic Constitution* (1988), Dr. Robert E. Svoboda writes:

> Ayurveda regards medicated enema as the most important purification method of all, because of the importance of the large intestine in health and disease. For example, the AIDS virus apparently first colonizes the colon and proliferates there before it floods the system. It can do so only if the colon is full of Ama to encourage it to grow. Medicated enemas eliminate pathogenic Ama and facilitate the absorption of Prana.

According to an article in the April 1991 *Longevity*, sales of Ayurvedic botanical products amount to at least $5 million annually. In a 1990 report on a study with rats, Maharishi proponent Hari M. Sharma, M.D., and associates conclude that *Maharishi Amrit Kalash*, administered as a food supplement, reduced both the incidence and number of breast tumors after chemically induced carcinogenesis. But the significance for humans is far from clear, and a number of medicinal plants of the traditional Ayurvedic pharmacopoeia have been shown to produce lesions of the liver and kidney.

In addition to carcinogens, the *Longevity* article cites as caveats the common use of a mercury salt in Ayurvedic preparations and poor quality control.

Maharishi Amrit Kalash costs about $95 for a month's supply. A 1991 MAPI flyer hails it as "food for perfection in life" and "the #1 protection against free radicals." It claims: "No other product contains so much of nature's wisdom compressed into one combination." Two formulations of the product, said to be "complementary," are available: *Ambrosia* (a tablet) and *Nectar* ("an herbal fruit concentrate"). *Ambrosia* allegedly promotes "vitality of body and mind" and "higher states of consciousness"; sixty Ambrosia tablets cost $45. The *Nectar* also is claimed to promote "higher states of consciousness"—by "creating a balanced physiology and an integrated functioning of body and mind." Eighteen ounces cost $50.

Maharishi Ayur-Veda products are not only prescribed by Ayurvedic physicians, but are marketed by mail and at health fairs. Magazine ads, for example, have invited readers to have their body type determined by completing a questionnaire and submitting it with $14.95 to MAPI, which responds with an analysis, "personalized dietary recommendations," and product literature. Similar questionnaires have been used at health fairs, where no fee is involved but the results are used as the basis for prescribing an herbal tea said to balance the person's doshas. The questions involve such characteristics as hair texture, mental activity, memory, size of teeth, type of dreams, and reactions to the weather. In the January/February 1991 *Nutrition Forum,* Dr. Stephen Barrett reported an amusing experience at the Ayur-Veda booth at Whole Life Expo in New York City:

> I was informed by a Maharishi Ayur-Veda exhibitor that my "doshas" were imbalanced, and he offered to sell me a tea to correct this. When I indicated that my health was good, he replied that achieving balance through Ayurvedic measures would prevent *future* trouble.

The Swami, the Doctor, and "Energy Medicine"

In 1991, I attended a "Conference on Clinical Nutrition" designed for chiropractors. It was held on June 8 and 9 at the Ritz-Carlton Hotel in Philadelphia, Pennsylvania, by the International College of Applied Kinesiology-USA following its five-day annual meeting. Applied kinesiology (AK) was concocted as a diagnostic method by chiropractor George

Goodheart in the mid-1960s. Goodheart theorized that muscle groups share "energy pathways" with internal organs. Testing muscles for relative strength and tone supposedly localizes illness by tapping the body's "innate intelligence." One of the goals of AK muscle-testing is to detect nutritional deficiencies and intolerance to specific foods. Probably several thousand chiropractors utilize AK.

Rudolph Ballentine, one of the speakers at the conference, was introduced as a graduate of Duke University and a former professor of psychiatry at Louisiana State University. He is also president of the Himalayan International Institute of Yoga Science and Philosophy of the U.S.A., in Honesdale, Pennsylvania. The institute's founder and spiritual head is Sri Swami Rama of the Himalayas, author of many yoga-related books, including *A Practical Guide to Holistic Health* (1980) and *Exercise Without Movement* (1984). The institute has twenty branches and affiliated centers across the United States and abroad. Ballentine is also director of the institute's Combined Therapy Program, which gives instruction to various patients in yoga and biofeedback, and he heads the Center for Holistic Medicine in New York City, which offers dietary counseling, biofeedback training, and shiatsu (Japanese acupressure). One of his books, *Transition to Vegetarianism* (1987), was favorably reviewed in the *American Journal of Clinical Nutrition*—a fact he made much of during his lecture.

Ballentine said he had been practicing "what amounts to general medicine for . . . almost twenty years, although . . . of a somewhat unusual type." After a residency in psychiatry, he "spent some time in India, studying Ayurveda and studying homeopathy. And that . . . changed the direction of my professional career, and my personal life, too." (The 1990 directory of the National Center for Homeopathy categorizes him as one who "practices homeopathy 75–100% of the time.")

"The first question that I want to deal with," he said, "is: Why should we bother to try to understand something about Ayurveda? . . . When I came back to the U.S. twenty years ago and started talking about Ayurveda, it drew a total blank. I mean, I would plan these lectures and nobody showed up. Nobody was interested, nobody knew what it was, and nobody wanted to know what it was. So, there's now a definite increase in awareness of the subject."

Yet, Ballentine stated three times that he felt "overwhelmed" by what he described as the huge, explosive outpouring of "holistic" treatments. "Out of three [holistic therapy] careers, I could maybe learn a few of the basic tools; and then, when will I have time to apply it all? So, you know, maybe I can get someone in my practice to help me [utilize] applied kinesiology. But, then, can we really communicate? [We'll] have to be able to coordinate our treatments."

Ballentine finally answered his own rhetorical question:

> Part of what we need is some kind of integrating conceptual scheme, something that will allow us to pull it all together.... And, you know, we're kind of unique in that we don't have that.... Other cultures, other societies, have what we call an indigenous system of medicine, some kind of conceptual framework that they use, that the person on the street uses to think about his health, and what he should eat, and what he should do for himself.... It's something that is common to almost every established culture in the world, but it doesn't exist here, and part of the reason is because we're a melting pot. And this is one of the things that sort of melted away and ran through the cracks.

He proposed Ayurveda as the agency of "a manageable conceptual scheme for individualizing and classifying patients." "The basic concept of disease," he said, can be understood best by "examining the level of functioning where energy flows" and by recognizing that "interruptions or irregularities or imbalances in that energy level of human functioning" are the key to understanding and correcting disease and ensuring longevity.

Ballentine described "energy medicine" as "the direction of the future. But we're really still kind of fumbling around how to understand it. And, you know, [there is] no need to reinvent the wheel. It doesn't mean the wheel can't be improved . . . but no need to invent it."

"Hoppy" Landings

On May 4, 1991, I interviewed a MAPI distributor and TM teacher at Newlife Expo '91 in New York City, a health symposium whose keynote speakers included macrobiotic guru Michio Kushi and leading iridology proponent Bernard Jensen, D.C.

> Q: Wouldn't you say a reading of the Vedas requires an esoteric, rather than an exoteric, approach?
> A: No. What it takes is, it takes somebody who knows what the Vedas truly are.
>
> Q: But what are the Vedas, in one sentence?
> A: They're like DNA. They're knowledge; they're pure knowledge. If they're properly read and properly understood, then you have the benefit of the Vedas.

Q: Can the same be said of the Bible?

A: I don't know. I'm not a biblical scholar.

Q: Do the Vedas represent all truth, or do they just contain grains of truth?

A: When people normally talk about the Vedas, they're thinking about the texts. But Veda, in true Vedanta [summaries in certain parts of the four Vedas that form the doctrinal basis of Hinduism], Veda is knowledge and it's not just what's in the texts; it's there at all times. The Vedas say this about themselves: . . . If you've got it together, we'll tell you what it's all about. . . . The Vedas are an external omnipresent reality just like the knowledge of DNA.

Q: I . . . read that the Maharishi . . . claimed that he could teach advanced meditators to fly. Does he still maintain this?

A: Oh, yes; oh, yes. In fact, I fly twice a day.

Q: When you say 'fly,' you mean physically fly?

A: Yeah, physically: the body lifts up off the ground.

Q: For how long did you stay off the ground?

A: Not long. . . . Patanjali [an ancient Hindu grammarian and exponent of yoga] . . . in the Vedantic text . . . says that there are different stages to flying. The first stage is just hopping. The next stage is hovering. The third and final stage is flying.

Q: And you are at what stage?

A: Hopping. And what has been found at two levels—one subjectively—is that there's a great feeling of bliss and exhilaration in the people who have learned this technique. They continue it for year after year because of that bliss. The second [level] is the objective measurement. There's an enormous amount of scientific literature showing that at the point of liftoff, there's an incredible coherence in the wave functioning aspects of awareness; and that's clearly indicated on electroencephalograms.

Q: Do you happen to know any meditators who have advanced to the third stage of flying?

A: No, no, no. Everyone seems to be at this hopping stage. Patanjali labored out that that will be how it progresses. It's a bit shallow to just talk about hopping if there's not someone who's standing from [the perspective of] the physics concept of the unified field. . . . I'll give you one real good example. . . . It's absolutely possible to take this pen, throw it on this hard table, and have it pop out the other side and fall to the ground. . . . On the quantum mechanical level of physics, it's a different ball game. Things aren't just as they seem on the classical Newtonian level. This technique—this yogic flying technique—begins to function from the quantum mechanical level of the mind.

Q: Do you follow an Ayurvedic diet?
A: Yes, but not rigidly. . . . The thing about Ayurvedic diet is, it's so very diverse. . . . It's not like you can't have ice cream. No, no, it's not like that. You just use your head, and in wintertime, you don't gobble lots of ice cream. . . . Every mother, if she'd just teach her child so that when they grow up, they'd just know that when you eat a meal, you don't eat as you're walking along—you sit, you eat, and sit after the meal for five-ten minutes, allow the food to digest, and then you can get up.

In the September/October 1991 issue of *Body, Mind, & Spirit*, freelance writer Barbara Rosen reports that the Maharishi has allegedly taught "yogic flying" to more than eighty thousand people around the world, and that competitions are held annually at local, national, and international levels. Rosen attended such a competition at the Los Angeles Transcendental Meditation Center in 1990 and says of the "yogic flyers": "In fact, they look like leaping frogs more than soaring eagles." She adds: "I must say I was a little disappointed in how it looked. . . . I could hear soft plops as they bounced along the foam padding."

"The reason I was disappointed in the spectacle," she explains, "is that the men looked like they were hopping with their muscles. It just didn't *look* like flying." She expressed this observation to a contestant, who responded: "The Wright Brothers are considered the pioneers of flying. Yet their first plane trips were only hops, too. That doesn't mean they weren't really flying." In 1987, a federal court jury awarded $137,890 to an ex-devotee who contended that TM organizations had falsely promised that he could learn to levitate, reduce stress, improve his memory, and reverse the aging process. According to the Spring 1992 *TM-EX Newsletter*, published by the Transcendental Meditation Ex-Members Support Group, the Maharishi responded in a telephone interview that "some planes fly, others don't," and said that the litigant had erred in "expecting too much." In 1988, an appeals court ordered a new trial. On June 20, 1991, the *Des Moines Register* reported that the case had been settled out of court for about $50,000.

In *Ayurveda and Immortality* (1986) "Vedic scientists" Scott Treadway, Ph.D., and Linda Treadway, Ph.D., expressed their esteem for the Maharishi and his programs. However, an interview in the September/

October 1992 *Spectrum* suggests a change of mind. The interviewer cited criticisms of Ayurveda and a television show "in which TM practitioners hopped around on mats, never getting more than twelve inches off the floor." Scott Treadway responded:

I think it's an unfortunate association with Ayurveda. There have been a lot of cult associations like that, especially when you're talking about a kind of exploitation by that kind of movement. They do it mainly for money, and I think that's unfortunate. Ayurveda is for mommies and not just swamis. . . . We certainly don't need to surrender to anyone, be dependent, bow down, worship, or pay too much to get it [Ayurveda]. . . . [We] will continue to push for the emancipation of Ayurveda beyond the personalities and people who want to latch onto Ayurveda for exploitation and greed.

Medicine or Cultism?

A long letter about Maharishi Ayur-Veda was published in the May 22/29, 1991 *Journal of the American Medical Association* (*JAMA*). Billed as a "Letter From New Delhi," it was co-authored by Deepak Chopra, Hari M. Sharma, and Brihaspati Dev Triguna. Unlike the others, Triguna, the only one located in New Delhi, is neither a medical doctor nor a physician by Western standards; he is a "pulse diagnostician." MAPI catalogs depict him with a halo.

In the letter, Chopra and his associates stated that anxiety and insomnia are caused by an "imbalance" of *vata*; anger, envy, and jealousy, by an imbalance of *pitta*; and greed and "feelings of attachment," by an imbalance of *kapha*. They called for "rigorous scientific investigation" of Maharishi Ayur-Veda. In August 1991, *JAMA* published a financial disclosure correction, which noted that each of the three had affiliations with Maharishi organizations that had not been disclosed with submission of their manuscript. *JAMA* followed through in its October 2, 1991 issue with an investigative report that was extremely critical of Ayurvedic claims and practices. The letters section of this issue contained twenty comments—pro and con—concerning the May 22/29 article. Chopra and two Ayurvedic organizations subsequently filed suit against the author of the report, the journal's editor, and the American Medical Association.

Meanwhile, the Natural Law Party was officially launched in April 1992 and fielded a presidential candidate and many candidates for state and federal offices. Its platform was expressed in a twenty-four-page advertisement, in tabloid format, distributed shortly before the November 1992 election. The health section stated:

> The Natural Law Party envisions a disease-free society, in which every American enjoys a long life in perfect health. By bringing life into accord with natural law, the prevention programs proposed by the Natural Law Party will eliminate disease and culture ideal health and vitality for everyone. . . .
>
> Research suggests that implementing the programs proposed by the Natural Law Party could cut healthcare costs in half, saving an estimated $400 billion annually for the nation.

The Bottom Line

Ayurveda proponents use a language of their own to describe practices that are not based upon the body of basic knowledge of health, disease, and health care that has been widely accepted by the scientific community. The Ayurvedic diet appears innocuous, but is based on religious, not scientific, principles.

7

What Price FAIM?
Vitalism Revisited

Addressing the "Needs of the Heart and Spirit"

The Foundation for the Advancement of Innovative Medicine (FAIM) is one of several politically active organizations whose raison d'être is the furtherance of vitalistic and other dubious therapies. In the Spring 1990 issue of *Innovation,* its quarterly newsletter, FAIM executive director and full-time lobbyist Monica Miller stated: "Contemporary alternative therapies build upon the interaction of the given therapy with the patient's life force. They observe the power of a meaningful life and address the needs of the heart and spirit. These therapies validate the individual through science and art."

FAIM defines innovative medicine as "a treatment or therapy of empirical benefit that is yet outside the mainstream of conventional medicine." Headquartered in Suffern, New York, the organization was formed in 1986 and incorporated in 1987 "as a voice for innovative medicine's professionals, physicians, patients, and suppliers." According to a 1991 symposium flyer:

> FAIM's mission is to secure free choice in health care. Our first goal is the development of a membership to serve as both a forum for exchange and a constituency for change. The second goal is to educate both those within the field and the general public as to the benefits and issues of innovative medicine. This activity includes the collection of statistical data with which to advocate our position. The third goal is guaranteed reimbursement for the

97

patients, be it through legislation, litigation or negotiation with state and insurance agencies. And lastly, in laying the groundwork for a climate receptive to medical innovation, we encourage research and development of promising new approaches.

The FAIM Educational Fund (FAIM ED) was incorporated in 1991. According to a 1992 symposium flyer, it "exists to promote the American health care consumer's access to information and education regarding health care alternatives." Its mission statement asserts: "Our final responsibility is to knowledge."

Articles in *Innovation* have promoted "alternative" cancer therapies, chelation therapy, homeopathy, shark cartilage for arthritis and for protection against tumor growth, and an oral bacterial preparation for chronic fatigue syndrome. One article describes how to sue insurance companies in small claims court when they deny claims for "complementary" treatment. Other articles blast fluoridation, mercury-amalgam fillings, and sugar (for allegedly causing digestive problems). A 1991 flyer urged members to ask their state legislators to support a bill to ensure that "unconventional" practitioners participate in the judging of practitioners accused of professional misconduct.

FAIM's *Directory of Professional Members* (1991) lists fifty-two healthcare practitioners, including twenty-five medical doctors, eight chiropractors, seven dentists, five osteopaths, three clinical psychologists, a psychotherapist, a certified social worker, a naturopath, and a nutritionist whose doctorate was awarded by Columbia Pacific University, an unaccredited correspondence school. All but one practice in New York State or New Jersey. The glossary (incorrectly) defines "allopathic medicine" as:

> The mainstream school of medicine whose therapeutic modalities are generally confined to surgery and synthetic drug therapies. Allopathic medicine utilizes the principle of opposites and is characterized by specialization according to diagnosis or anatomy. All licensed M.D.s have a basic education in allopathic medicine.

During 1992, FAIM's board of trustees consisted of eight medical doctors and one dentist, all of whom practiced within New York State. The board's president—and a FAIM co-founder—is Robert C. Atkins, M.D., author of *Dr. Atkins' Diet Revolution* (1971), *Dr. Atkins' Superenergy Diet* (1977), *Dr. Atkins' Nutrition Breakthrough* (1981), *Dr. Atkins' Health Revolution* (1988), and *Dr. Atkins' New Diet Revolution* (1992). Atkins is also president of the New York County Chapter of the New York State

Society of Homeopathic Medicine. In the press release promoting his *Health Revolution*, he stated: "There is only one disease which is called imbalance, and it is combated by the restoration of balance, which is another word for health." He says that, "Nutrition has been useful in just about every condition I have treated," and claims that it is difficult or impossible to conduct double-blind tests of the "alternative" methods he espouses. In an interview reported in the January 1992 issue of Swanson Health Products' *Health Shopper*, Atkins stated that orthodox doctors "deliberately define quackery as using unprovens. Then they create standards of proof that only moneyed corporations can afford." In another interview, reported in *Challenging Orthodoxy* (1991), he stated:

> I'm really critical of the scientist who believes that the double-blind is an appropriate modality to screen out certain types of doctor-patient interrelationships. I feel that as medical philosophers that's a flawed conclusion. Throughout the history of mankind, the effectiveness of a doctor in healing a patient depended on a relationship between the healer and the healee. And, for the healer to be effective, he has got to believe that he is a healer. He really, in essence, has got to believe that whatever he's got in there works.

Atkins founded and directs The Atkins Centers for Complementary Medicine in New York City, which recently moved into a modern six-story building. He also publishes *The Atkins Health Letter* and hosts "Design for Living," a nightly radio talk show on station WOR. The former host of the program was Carlton Fredericks, who, in the mid-1980s, performed "nutritional consultations" costing $200 at Atkins's offices. Fredericks had virtually no training in scientific nutrition, but made a career of recommending nutritional remedies for the gamut of disease. In 1945 he pled guilty to practicing medicine without a license after New York State authorities found he was diagnosing illnesses and prescribing vitamins. Thereafter, until his association with Atkins, he confined his advice to books, lectures, and his radio talk show. A heavy smoker, Fredericks died of a heart attack in 1987 at the age of seventy-three.

In an interview in the March 1991 issue of Swanson Health Products' *Health Shopper*, Atkins defined complementary medicine as a synthesis of orthodox and "alternative" medicine integrating "the best of both." The services under his auspices include acupuncture, chiropractic, homeopathy, bioenergetics, clinical ecology, chelations, ozone therapy, neurolinguistic programming, ultraviolet blood irradiation, and "an assortment of unclassified techniques." According to a form letter sent to a prospective patient as part of a questionnaire packet in 1991, this "diverse mixture of healing arts" has "a single common denominator: all are safer modalities than those in common medical usage." Atkins further contends that, "Any valid healing art used on behalf of an individual can have an additive benefit when combined with other valid healing arts," and that, "The greater the number of valid systems used, the greater the probability of success." The questionnaire packet included the Atkins Health Indicator Test, which covers such symptoms as: constant tiredness, hunger between meals or at night, depression, awakening after a few hours' sleep, fearfulness, indecisiveness, insecurity or poor self-image, moodiness, feeling "like crying inside," making "mountains out of molehills," reduced initiative, boredom, bad dreams, and reduced sex drive.

A "Complementary Medicine" Smorgasbord

Each year, FAIM sponsors several symposia featuring prominent practitioners of "alternative" medicine. On January 26 and 27, 1991, I attended the first of the year's series at the New York Penta Hotel (now the Ramada Hotel), across the street from Madison Square Garden. About five hundred people attended the two Saturday sessions, and about four hundred attended the single Sunday session. Virtually all were white and appeared older than forty.

As I entered the eighteenth-floor hall, I spied what I hoped was a coffee urn, and shortly made my way toward it. But I discovered disappointedly that the urn contained an herbal tea marketed by Sunrider International, one of about seventeen companies with booths in the back of the hall. At the Sunrider booth, I paid $2.00 for a 1.5-ounce confection called *SunBar*—an "herb food" containing water lily bulb, Chinese asparagus root, and several other exotic ingredients, with sorbitol as its primary coating ingredient. The product tasted medicinal and was so hard and adhesive I feared it might loosen my mercury-amalgam fillings. As I chewed apprehensively, the Sunrider salesman introduced me to another distributor—said to be a registered dietitian with a master's degree in nutrition—who expressed antipathy toward double-blind studies. Other exhibitors at the symposium included the following.

- The Atkins Centers for Complementary Medicine, which markets "Dr. Atkins' Targeted Nutrition Program." This is a supplementation regimen in which "building blocks" are added to a "basic formula" to "help the body create its own cures." The seventeen "building blocks" include *Anti-Arthritic Formula, Cardiovascular Formula, Diabetes Mellitus Formula, Heart Rhythm Formula, Hypoglycemia Formula,* and *Urinary Frequency Formula.* (The labels of some of these products do not contain the full name of the product but merely a code—such as *CV* for *Cardiovascular Formula* and *DM* for *Diabetes Mellitus Formula.*) A brochure states that the formulas evolved over twenty-five years of Atkins's experience in using nutrition to treat more than forty thousand patients. The supplements are sold at a counter in the lobby of his office building.

• Boericke & Tafel, Inc., in Santa Rosa, California, which calls itself "America's oldest homeopathic pharmaceutical firm." Its *Alfalfa Tonic* was promoted at the meeting "for symptomatic relief of insomnia and nervous stress."

• Great Smokies Diagnostic Laboratory, in Asheville, North Carolina, which performs a variety of nonstandard tests. Its flyer encourages people to ask their doctor about the lab's Comprehensive Digestive Stool Analysis (CSDA): "Discover How Much Valuable Information Lies Hidden in Your Stool Sample!" The flyer further states: "The CSDA now detects levels of Short Chain Fatty Acids. Low levels of some of these may be associated with increased risk of colon cancer and ulcerative colitis."

• Health from the Sun, in Newton Upper Falls, Massachusetts, which markets *Sanhelios* herb products, including *Circu Caps, Prosta Caps, Circu Balm, Kalm Caps,* and *The 3-Day Diet*—"a 'near fast' diet for losing 7 to 10 pounds in 3 days."

• Huggins Diagnostic Center, in Colorado Springs, Colorado, which says it is "the leader in diagnosing and treating patients who suffer from mercury toxicity due to dental amalgam." Its brochure recommends hair analysis—to detect supposed mercury toxicity—and sequential removal of mercury-amalgam fillings. It also advertises electrolyte replacement beverages, including *Jungle Juice.* A flyer available at the booth states in bold red letters: "You wouldn't take your child's temperature with a leaky thermometer."

• Klabin Marketing in New York City, which markets *Aloe-Ace*— "whole leaf" aloe vera juice from "organically grown" aloe vera leaves, complete with sap, rind, and gel. According to George Klabin, the sap and rind contain an immune stimulant, and several hundred "important healing elements" have been identified in the leaf.

• Natren, Inc., of North Hollywood, California, which featured *Bulgaricum I.B.*, a *Lactobacillus bulgaricum* culture that allegedly "aids in the production of white blood cells" and "activates the immune system."

• Ocean Health Products, which distributed flyers suggesting that shark cartilage is effective against cancer, diabetic retinopathy, osteoarthritis, psoriasis, and various other conditions. A flyer written by FAIM board member Ronald Hoffman, M.D., states: "Although there have been no clinical tests performed, several doctors and chiropractors have noticed that when used regularly, shark cartilage seems to reduce the incidence of muscle pulls, inflamed joints, and stiffness due to injury." Hoffman, who practices in New York City, also publishes a newsletter and sells supplements.

• Tachyon International of Fort Lee, New Jersey, which marketed *Tachyon Cells* and *Tachyon Water*— "Phenomena of the 90's New From Japan!!" Tachyons are purely hypothetical particles postulated to travel faster than light and backward in time. Experiments conducted to determine whether they exist have come out negative, and nearly all physicists doubt their existence. But according to Tachyon International's flyer, tachyons have not only been discovered and characterized, but "extracted" and turned to practical use. How was this done? A reprint distributed at Newlife Expo '91 describes the method as "the inventor's secret." The flyer states that the tachyon "possesses a nature which goes beyond the conventional terms of physics" and is equivalent to *Ch' i* or *ki* in the Orient. It further states that the Tachyon Research Association has succeeded in charging various substances with tachyon energy. The product *Tachyon Cells*— pads said to contain tachyon-charged "cells"—is one example. The flyer quotes testimonials asserting that the pads—which are to be taped to the skin—are effective for wrenched, frozen, or painful shoulders, swollen knees, and "abnormal coldness." In the March/April 1992 *Newlife*, naturopath David Blodgett offers his own testimonial on tachyon energy and writes: "The tachyon seems to act as a catalyst and balance for the life energy and healing process, with no side effects or contra-indications." He concludes: "The time has finally come when we can begin to replace drugs with energy for healing."

"Looked Like He Was Cured"

I took a front seat before the "festivities" began at the FAIM symposium. To my left sat a pathologically obese man whose name badge indicated he was a dentist and whose behavior suggested narcolepsy. On my right, an elderly woman eyed my note-taking suspiciously while she gabbed about root canals, Atkins's radio program, and a turkey sandwich she had bought at a GNC store that morning.

On both days, the symposium program kicked off with welcoming remarks from Atkins, whom Monica Miller introduced as "our guiding light." Atkins, who looked overweight, said that "freedom of choice" in matters of health should be a major political issue. "When we get our potentially terminal illness, or when we get an illness which is going to be able to debilitate us, this," he said, "is where we need to be able to make that intelligent choice. Now the reason that we don't have freedom of choice is that there are too many people in our country that don't even perceive that there are other choices." He ascribed this "lack of awareness" to the reliance of the media and politicians on physicians "connected with some trade organization such as the American Medical Association."

Atkins stated that FAIM may be growing so rapidly, "it will become the predominant organization in the country for the principle of freedom of choice." Then he complained about pressure placed on the nutritional supplement industry and about FDA "Gestapo raids" to enforce labeling laws.

He related the story of a fifty-three-year-old man with lung cancer who had recently gone to Memorial Sloan-Kettering Cancer Center, where he had been offered only one mode of therapy: radiation. Atkins said he had subsequently offered the man at least twenty treatment options, "all from the field of complementary medicine, all of them using a different model." The next day, Atkins declared, the man "looked like he was cured." Atkins did not say whether he had treated the patient, but he implied that the patient's improved appearance had reflected a change in attitude—the result of his having introduced hope. The aim of cancer therapy, he suggested, should be to "just treat the underlying condition—the terrain." He then said that perhaps a "new medical science called 'terrainology'. . . should be our new banner."

Atkins exhorted the attendees to scout and recruit new members, estimating FAIM's membership at 1,600. "I'm looking for ten thousand by the end of 1991. I want to show that growth pattern to the politicians. I want . . . people [to] recognize that here is a political force . . . to be reckoned with." Then he solicited volunteers for a membership expansion committee. But in September 1992, I called FAIM and was informed that its membership was about 2,400. Later I learned that Monica Miller had left FAIM to launch an umbrella group called the People's Consortium for Medical Freedom.

The Prime-Rib Rubdown

The first talk, on "Women's Health," was delivered by Christiane Northrup, M.D., a clinical assistant professor of obstetrics and gynecology at the University of Vermont, past-president of the American Holistic Medical Association, and co-founder of "Women to Women," a women's health-care center in Yarmouth, Maine. She had contributed to *Doctors Look at Macrobiotics* (1988).

Northrup alluded to studies "now showing that mind is the result of consciousness" and that "consciousness creates the body." She described the immune system as "a liquid mind . . . affected by everything—colors, light, vitamins, brown rice." She advised us to think of ourselves as holograms. Health is "not just about food," she emphasized. "I tell people if they're going to have a prime rib, get a massage; maybe it'll cancel . . . out [the prime rib]." Later she stated: "When you have emotions that remain locked in your body, which you do not feel, your need for vitamins is increased."

"Men's and women's physical energy is completely different," she asserted, likening male energy to "heaven's force" and female energy to "earth's energy coming upward . . . into the vagina." She also said that the chakras correspond to the major endocrine organs. (In yoga philosophy, the chakras are centers of spiritual energy in the human body.) "The uterus is in the second chakra," she told us, which is "symbolic of relationships, creativity, and security."

Northrup attributed the high incidence of breast cancer in Maine to insufficient sunlight, and fibroid uterus and endometriosis partly to "blocked energy in the pelvis." She said that therapeutic touch accompanies the endometrial biopsies she performs. Premenstrual syndrome, she asserted, often recurs if women don't "get in touch with what their mission is here on the planet."

Treating Invisible Cancers

Atkins introduced the next speaker, Harvey Bigelsen, M.D., as "the first professor of terrainology . . . politically, a most important figure to us . . .

the man who single-handedly got the first significant bill [passed] enabling M.D.s who had another approach to have the protection of homeopathic boards [in] Arizona, the most conservative state in the country." Bigelsen, the director of the Center for Progressive Medicine in Phoenix, Arizona, described himself as a "trained ophthalmologist" who had been in the field of "holistic" medicine for fifteen years. "Traditional medicine," he declared, "made no sense to me whatsoever," because:

> There was no known reason for disease. . . . There's no rhyme or reason whatsoever to disease. . . . The treatment for the cause and the cure of chronic disease is a 100 percent failure. . . . That frustrates me. I'm a scientist.

Bigelsen said that thanks to the passage of the above-mentioned bill, he has been "allowed . . . to do things that other places couldn't do. . . . My work can be done in the open completely. For the past ten years, I've been on television out in Arizona, and the establishment cannot do anything about it."

He claimed that the length of time an unstained drop of blood "lives" on a microscope slide is an indication of the health of the patient from whom it was drawn. He said his basic philosophy is that "there is a harmony in this universe." Bigelsen also claimed that everyone harbors the "spore form" of cancer in 20 percent of the body's cells. "Twenty percent is fine," he assured us. But cancer is on the increase, he said, "because of the tremendous pollution of the . . . internal terrain of the body." According to Bigelsen, cancer is a contagious, "transferable" mold, and is not spread via the bloodstream or lymphatic system. He said he was treating approximately 40 to 60 percent of his patients for cancer, but that these patients didn't know they were being treated for cancer. "They will have it in five to ten years if I don't fix them now," he explained. He further claimed that HIV is not "necessarily" the cause of AIDS but is an "inhabitant" of the disease.

Cancer: "Nature's Verdict"?

Next, Atkins introduced Mark Anderson, co-author of *Empty Harvest*, as "the authority on the subject of what has gone wrong with our planet." Anderson's lecture was titled "How Agricultural Practices Rob You of Health." "What we have in today's world," he lamented, "is a health-disease paradigm built upon a pharmaceutical-chemical approach [from] which nutritional concepts can't get out. Nutritional insights and understanding find a difficulty in being expressed." Anderson likened white bread to money without precious metal backing. He stated:

> This discussion on nutrition gives one the impression that the whole issue can be settled by making the right choices in the supermarket. And it ain't so. I don't care how informed you are. ... The laws of the universe say you can't make something out of nothing.

He produced a soil sample and declared: "Soil is what makes human beings healthy, because soil is what makes plants healthy. Plants don't grow in supermarkets." He called modern farming "the art of killing" and further stated: "If the food was organically grown, it's not the fact that it lacks pesticides that's so important: it's the fact that the food survived without pesticides. That means the farmer had to invest his skills, time, and money into regenerating, revitalizing, the basis of plant growth—soil, not oil."

Having referred earlier to Bigelsen's description of cancer as a mold, Anderson stated that such fungi living in the human body yield "nature's verdict upon the quality of health of our tissue. If it is hungry, starved, and diseased, it deserves to be attacked." He explained: "Bacteria and fungus are not the enemy. They are just showing us that we are deficient. Consequently, they are cleaning us out, removing the dying, weak, necrotic tissue. This is the great failure of the germ theory of medicine."

Waxing mystical, Anderson said that "whatever happens anywhere, happens everywhere, eventually. ... This is the global consciousness of personal health, that my health is inexorably linked to what is happening as the forests of Tibet are cut down." He pronounced vitamins "the greatest health discovery of the twentieth century," because they had "finally proved that there was a cause of health."

"Artificial chemical fertilizers," Anderson concluded, "are the great seduction of the twentieth century that have led to the ruination of the human species."

Suicide and Mercury Amalgams

Hal Huggins, D.D.S., lectured on "Amalgams and Root Canals." He stated that if "negative-current" fillings are removed first, the patient gets better, but if "positive-current" fillings are removed first, the patient gets worse; "and the reason for that is so obvious, I'm not going to bother to go into it with you."

Huggins stated that dental diseases include "the incurables and the unexplained," such as chest pains, depression, and suicidal ideation. For "calcium imbalances," he said he prescribes not calcium supplementation but massage therapy. He said the two psychologists on his staff were very important because "when you take out the fillings, you start releasing people's emotional problems." Suicide, he declared, "is such a big part of the amalgam issue." He also claimed that root canals are dangerous and that he has seen dramatic improvement in patients after the removal of teeth containing root canals. He admitted he couldn't explain this alleged improvement, but said that acupuncture meridians might be involved.

"Father Earth" Panics

Atkins said he had chosen the next speaker—Michael Weiner, Ph.D.—because "herbal medicine is every bit as important as nutritional medicine as one of the cornerstones of complementary medicine." He stated that Weiner had received his doctorate, in "Nutritional Ethnomedicine," from the University of California at Berkeley. "And when they found out what he did with it," Atkins added, "they decided they were never going to issue another one—because what he did with it was create an herbal revolution." Weiner also holds M.S. and M.A. degrees in medical botany and medical anthropology from the University of Hawaii. He is the author of fifteen books, including *Weiner's Herbal* (1982), and co-author of *The Complete Book of Homeopathy* (1981). Like Atkins, Weiner hosts a radio talk show—"Dr. Weiner's Herb and Nutrition Hour"—on station WOR. He is a spokesperson for Twinlab, of Ronkonkoma, New York, and "director of scientific affairs" for Nature's Herbs, of Orem, Utah. Both companies sponsor the radio program.

Weiner told us: "Much of what you have learned to incorporate in your life is already in the scientific literature. It is just not promulgated by your healer, in general." "Trial and error," he said, "is an incredible system, because if [a treatment] works, it tends to be used over and over again. If it kills the patient, it's not used any more.... I wish some of the people using chemotherapeutic agents used trial and error." The audience applauded.

Later he stated he had been taking "megadoses of many nutrients, particularly vitamin C" for twenty years. He had been "converted to vitaminology ... by many leaders in the field," including his "granddaddy" Linus Pauling. Nevertheless, about three weeks earlier, he said, "I—Father Earth himself—got sick. Isn't that terrible." He said that when vitamin therapy had proved ineffective, he had panicked slightly. But, he claimed, as a consequence of taking one capsule of a particular herb, his flu had disappeared instantly.

(Pauling himself has been taking huge doses of vitamin C daily for many years. Recently, after discovering that he has prostate cancer, he claimed that his vitamin C intake had delayed the cancer's onset for twenty years.)

"Inject the Stuff"

Let's Live columnist Jonathan V. Wright, M.D., shared his "Pearls from a Complementary Physician's Notebook," sounding short of breath throughout his talk. He recommended *The National Enquirer* as a source of medical information.

"One of the things that we like to know about," he said, "if we happen to have a cancer and we're undergoing any sort of a treatment is: How am I doing? Of course, those of us who are in deep touch with our bodies might be able to tell that without any sort of a test"—indeed, might be "in touch enough not to [have developed] cancer in the first place."

Wright cited "an old principle in nutritional and orthomolecular medicine": "If you think a nutrient ought to work . . . and it isn't working . . . before you give it up, inject the stuff." After Wright finished, Atkins praised him for being open-minded, dedicated, and original.

(Wright evidently practices what he preaches. FAIM's first 1992 newsletter reported that FDA officials, teamed with local police, had searched Wright's offices and seized various injectable vitamins and other products that the agency considered misbranded or mislabeled. "Alternative" practitioners and the health-food industry are very upset about the raid.)

"I Treat the Blood"

The Saturday afternoon session concluded with a panel discussion moderated by Michael B. Schachter, M.D., vice president of FAIM and a laetrile enthusiast. When a woman asked Weiner if one can overdose on herbs, he replied that trial and error is "the only commonsense approach because we are going into areas that do not have . . . extensive documentation."

Schachter asked Bigelsen what kinds of "therapeutic maneuvers" he uses to treat his patients. Bigelsen responded: "I treat the blood, not necessarily the patient." (How unholistic!) The offerings he reported include the introduction of "debris-eating germs" into the bloodstream, injections of lactic acid to stimulate metabolism, "fetal cell therapy," and "scar therapy," which includes injections into circumcision scars. "You gotta get the pollution out of the body," he explained.

A question regarding the diagnosis of "mercury toxicity" was put to Dr. Huggins, who replied with a description of a no-win predicament:

> If the urinary excretion of mercury is very low, then we figure the patient has "retention toxicity"—that is, they're retaining the mercury. If the hair [analysis] shows very low levels of mercury, then this also [indicates] retention toxicity. . . . The low levels of mercury are the ones that scare me a lot more than the high levels.

Later he clarified his position: "The only time we really recommend removing of amalgams is for people who are interested in their health."

When to Consult a Quack

"Once you have gotten the satisfaction of seeing your patients get well," Atkins said in his welcoming address at the Sunday session, "you can't go back to an inferior brand of medicine, which is my name for conventional medicine. I hate to say it, but conventional medicine just doesn't measure up."

Pat McGrady, Jr., was the first lecturer on Sunday. His talk was titled "The Cancer Patient's Right to Live." Atkins said that McGrady "has the broadest fund of knowledge about alternatives which are available to the cancer patient . . . than anyone I've ever encountered." He described McGrady as a best-selling author and operator of a "referral service" for cancer patients (CANHELP). In 1991, McGrady's reports cost $400.

"If you've played any role in [a] personal war against cancer," McGrady said, "you know that the cancer patient has two enemies: the disease itself and those who exploit this war for their own gain." He stated that the latter enemy may be the more formidable, including "do-good" societies, the FDA, the National Cancer Institute, and the American Medical Association. "There is no substitute for freedom of medical choice," McGrady declared. "It's as important as religion or speech. We *should* try to eliminate quackery, but most of it is government-sponsored." He further claimed that new and experimental methods within scientific medicine have no track record and are unlikely to develop any.

McGrady said his business is to find therapies for clients that "offer them a chance of extending their survival and improving their quality of life." He stated that he talks to 2,000 cancer patients annually. He advised: "Stay away from the quacks in general, but if your kid has a brain cancer, send him to one." He said of cancer surgery: "The ultimate twitches of the scalpel often produce a grotesque mutilation making a human being almost unrecognizable as such. Many doctors never learn."

In the November 1991 issue of *Probe,* investigative reporter David Zimmerman analyzed a report that CANHELP had prepared for a friend of his with a virulent form of lung cancer. The report, said Zimmerman, included

> 11 single-space pages of chatty but confusing information on alternative treatments, interspersed with news and press release data about conventional therapists, and information on some cancer specialists who fall between the two schools. Highly recommended . . . is a regimen that requires a restrictive diet, the swallowing of 100 to 150 or more pills each day . . . and coffee enemas.

Perhaps more important, Zimmerman observed, McGrady's report overlooked a promising new treatment whose results had not yet been published in a scientific journal, but which were readily available to physicians and the public from the National Cancer Institute's information services.

Zimmerman concluded that McGrady, though well-intentioned, was "trying to practice some form of medicine, by mail and telephone, which we believe he is not equipped for, or professionally trained to do."

"Magnetic" Personalities

Next, during a time slot designated "New Health Products," several exhibitors came forward to promote their wares. Kunio Yanagida, a Japanese man representing Tachyon International, claimed that tachyon energy can be extracted from the atmosphere with a "special device" and used to: (1) power motor vehicles and electric shavers, (2) recharge batteries, (3) turn regular cigarettes into "light" versions, and (4) improve athletic performance.

William Philpott, M.D., a proponent of "magnetic field therapy," was the symposium's last speaker. Atkins introduced him as "a physician with a nationwide constituency." Philpott said he had practiced medicine for forty years before retiring in May 1989. He revealed that he had had a fundamentalist Christian upbringing, had majored in theology, and had apparently been destined to be a preacher. Philpott claimed that 70 percent of human energy comes from food and that most of the remaining 30 percent comes from the earth's magnetic field. He added that "tachyon energy" is a very important source of energy for humans. He professed that one can "accentuate" the magnetic field through which the blood flows, and thus have "more energy," by following a practice he maintains daily: keeping a magnet in a pocket over the heart. He further recommended sleeping with a magnet at the crown of the head. Philpott is co-author of *Biomagnetic Handbook: A Guide to Medical Magnetics, The Energy Medicine of Tomorrow* (1990). His company, Enviro-Tech Products, of Choctaw, Oklahoma, sells a large variety of magnets whose "suitability for a particular use must be determined by the buyer."

The "Paranoid Announcement"

On October 26, 1991, I visited FAIM again at its third and last symposium of the year, which took place in the Grand Ballroom of the Omni Park Central Hotel in New York City. The nineteen exhibitors included twelve companies concerned with nutrient supplements, herbal preparations, homeopathic remedies, and/or Anthroposophical products. Also represented were: American Biologics, "hospital and world leader in enzyme therapy"; the Fertility Awareness Center, "promoting Pre-choice, the natural way"; R & S Organics, marketing a variety of minimally processed snacks; *Raum & Zeit*, a periodical focused on "alternative methods of medicine and physics"; Vaccination Alternatives, "promoting informed choice concerning vaccination and immunization"; and ACT UP (AIDS Coalition to Unleash Power), an activist group fighting for "freedom of health choice." One of the exhibitors, Weleda Inc. of Spring Valley, New York, is affiliated with an Anthroposophical center called the Threefold Community, and produces and distributes skin-care products and homeopathic formulas based on "indications" given by Rudolf Steiner. FAIM's Saturday program included presentation of a Weleda film on Anthroposophical remedies. Another exhibitor, Multi-Pure Corporation, markets water purification systems and *Stop Drops II*, "the new, improved, all natural, homeopathic, herbal, fast acting, fabulous Appetite Control Drops," according to a letter distributed at the symposium. *Stop Drops II* is said to be an alternative to a "strict diet-exercise program.... demanding, tough, restrictive and frankly boring"—the "old" way to lose weight.

Serafina Corsello, M.D., secretary of FAIM and a former orthomolecular psychiatrist, acted as chairperson. "These symposiums," she said, "have become a beacon of knowledge and an opportunity for you, the public, and us, the medical practitioners, to get together and share ideas. We are bound by a fierce desire for advancement of knowledge and freedom of choice. This bond will make our dream a reality, or so I hope." Between the first lecture and a question-and-answer session, she stated:

> Why do we punish people for being innovative in this country? . . . I now must make a paranoid announcement: Any member of any governmental agency—NCI [National Cancer Institute], FDA, or the like—that is here must stand up and announce himself or herself. . . . according to the law. We have been spied [on] before. We have evidence that they come here to spy [on] us. The law states they must stand up and announce themselves. Stand or leave.

As no one stood or left, Corsello said: "Okay? There's nobody. So, they don't know what we're doing." Then she asked our forgiveness, but added that she would make this "paranoid announcement" from time to time "to protect us and our speakers."

"Trusting Our Own Judgment"

In the Spring 1990 issue of *The Atkins Health Letter*, Atkins announced that FAIM's professional members had set up a legal defense fund "for doctors unfairly put upon for their honorable practice of alternative medicine." Noting that FAIM member Warren M. Levin, M.D., faced disciplinary action by the New York State Department of Health Board of Professional Conduct, Atkins appealed for donations:

> The only charge is that Dr. Levin uses the time-honored techniques of alternative treatment: there are sixty charges under that heading. There is no question that I employ the same or equivalent practices.
> If the orthodox majority prevails in the matter of Dr. Levin, then this will be a signal that they can take away the license of any doctor who they may not like. . . .
> The next doctor you save may be your own.

In July 1991, Atkins testified for Levin before the Board of Professional Conduct and was asked how practitioners of "complementary medicine" judge whether a therapy is trustworthy. He replied:

We do have our own groups, and we do have our own peer-review meetings. We even have our peer-reviewed literature, which I must say is lagging behind because only a small percentage of the complementary physicians have been able to find the time to write. . . .

I listen carefully to my colleagues who make a suggestion, and then I begin to try it out until I have done something which doctors through the ages have done. They have arrived at their own conclusions based on their own experience.

I think it is very difficult to assume that a doctor can do that, but yet all of us in complementary medicine have arrived at our conclusions basically by trusting our own judgment, based on the accumulation of experience which is both first-hand, second-hand, and from the literature.

In September 1992, the board found Levin guilty of "gross negligence," "fraudulent practice," and "moral unfitness" and recommended that his license be revoked. The board's final report stated:

Respondent has a litany of unproven and medically unnecessary tests that he runs on virtually all patients. He uses these tests—whatever their results may be—to convince his patients that his unconventional kinds of treatment are necessary. Many of the tests . . . have no clinical validity, are not appropriate general diagnostic procedures . . . or are unnecessary.

Respondent employs a number of treatment modalities of unproven value. His nutritional therapy utilizes megadoses of many vitamins, minerals, and supplements. . . . In addition to being of dubious efficacy, these substances are not innocuous. Further, the financial cost to the patient is significant.

In December 1992, a federal grand jury accused Harvey Bigelson, M.D., of one count of conspiracy to defraud the United States; sixty-three counts of false, fictitious, or fraudulent claims; forty-four counts of mail fraud; one count of conspiracy to commit an offense against the United States; and eight counts of obstruction of proceedings before departments, agencies and committees. The indictment states that he attempted to collect about $8,000 for colonic therapy, massage therapy, and chiropractic services (including acupuncture)—which he knew were not covered under Medicare—by submitting claim forms on which they were represented by procedure code numbers for services covered under "physical medicine." The indictment also charges that Bigelson and two associates attempted to evade prosecution by changing data in the computer account histories of

several patients and by submitting altered and falsified progress notes in
response to a grand jury subpoena.

The Bottom Line: Innovation or Nonsense?

Drs. Petr Skrabanek and James McCormick write in *Follies and Fallacies
in Medicine* (1990):

> The claims of systems of alternative medicine all have two things
> in common. They have no detectable or coherent raison d'etre
> other than the enthusiasm of their advocates and, almost without
> exception, they claim to cure or alleviate a very large number of ill-
> defined and quite disparate ills.

True scientists regard innovation as a potential springboard for
studies that can lead to proof, disproof, or alternate hypotheses. FAIM is
using it only as a political catchword.

8

The "Weird Science" of Anthroposophy

"Baby Science"

The Fall 1991 *Skeptical Inquirer* provides the following account of "weird science" taught at the San Francisco Waldorf School, part of a system founded in 1919 by occultist Rudolf Steiner (1861-1925). The father of a prospective student attended an open house at the school and concluded that the teachers were highly dedicated and that the teaching methods were very progressive. He enrolled his son in the sixth grade. Later, however, he discovered that one of Steiner's books sold at the school included the statement: "If the blonds and blue-eyed people died out, the human race will become increasingly dense if men do not arrive at a form of intelligence that is independent of blondness." Then the boy complained that he was being taught "baby science," in which the elements were said to be earth, air, fire, and water. The father examined several lesson books, in which "planetary influences" were said to affect plant growth and the body was said to consist of "the nerve-sense system, the metabolic-muscular system, and the rhythmic system." He further discovered that the science curriculum was based entirely on empiricism—observation without regard to theory. He attempted to organize a parents' committee to reform the science curriculum, but his proposal was met with disinterest. Then his request for a hearing with the school's administration was turned down, and a delegation of teachers threatened his family with expulsion. Defeated, he withdrew his son from the school.

115

"Occult Wisdom"

Anthroposophy is not a user-friendly philosophy. Tortuous and dense, even forbidding, it is the most occult of the systems explored in this book. It provides no short cuts to comprehension, and at once defies simplification and tempts oversimplification.

Anthroposophy sprouted in the soil of Theosophy (also called Theosophism). "Theosophy" is derived from the Greek words for "god" (*theos*) and "wisdom" (*sophy*). Uncapitalized, it refers to any religious system claiming that mystical insight into God's nature is attainable, and may be thought of as "speculative mysticism." Capitalized, however, the term signifies the composite of Hindu, Buddhist, cabalistic, Neo-Platonic, and Gnostic elements embedded in the tenets of the Theosophical Society. Although not directly concerned with diet or nutrition, Theosophy seems to constitute much of the bedrock of paranormal nutrition. During my "spiritual quest," described briefly in Chapter 1, Theosophy impressed me as a wonderful bastion of esoteric knowledge.

The Theosophical Society was co-founded in New York in 1875 by the mysterious Madame Helena Petrovna Blavatsky (1831-1891), who liked to be called "HPB." Born in the Ukraine, she allegedly had psychic powers and the ability to perceive nonphysical beings during her childhood. As an adult, she weighed over two hundred pounds, smoked cigars, and was wont to use bawdy language.

In *The Key to Theosophy*, HPB explained that Theosophy is "Divine Knowledge or Science" derived from a philosophical system whose primary object is "to inculcate certain great moral truths" upon disciples and all "lovers of the truth." Its chief aim, she wrote, is to reconcile all religions, sects, and nations under a common system of ethics, based on eternal truths. As head of the Theosophical Society, HPB effected such "miracles" as "spirit rappings" and "astral bells" to muster converts, but fraud was detected on several occasions. She professed to communicate telepathically with godlike personages called "the Masters" or "the Mahatmas," three of whom she identified as the real founders of the society. Her first book, *Isis Unveiled* (1877), occupies more than 1,300 pages. In *The Occult Underground* (1974), James Webb labels its style "appalling" and describes it as a "magpie-like accumulation of mysticism, tall stories and archaeology," with a vicious anti-Christian bias." Yet HPB's personality was so enthralling that she made numerous converts, even among the native inhabitants of India, a country mired in firmly established spiritual traditions. Headquartered there today, the Theosophical Society has about thirty-five thousand members.

Time-Life Books' *Ancient Wisdom and Secret Sects* states that the Theosophical Society became:

> in effect a great cultural funnel through which much of the occult wisdom of the ancients and of the East was collected and passed on to twentieth-century Western civilization. More than any other single entity, the society was responsible for discovering and reviving interest in the mystic arts and beliefs that later were taken up by adherents of the New Age, ranging from astral travel to Zen and encompassing astrology, reincarnation, karma, gurus and swamis, transcendental meditation, vegetarianism, and a general attitude of acceptance of the supernatural.

Rudolf Steiner: "Scientific Seer" or Mad Scientist?

Rudolf Steiner, called a "Scientific Seer" by *MD* magazine in 1969, was born in 1861 to Austrian parents in Kraljevic, which was then in Austro-Hungary, later in Yugoslavia. His father was a railway clerk and wanted him to become a railway civil engineer. By the age of eight, Steiner is said to have experienced clairvoyance, including perception of the spirit of a dead relative. He is also said to have perceived the "invisible energies" of plants. His family eventually settled near Vienna, where, at the age of fifteen, he supposedly met an herbalist who taught him the occult lore of plants. When he was nineteen, the herbalist allegedly introduced him to a spiritual adept known only as "the Master," who initiated Steiner into the occult tradition. Steiner reportedly learned from "the Master" that his life's "spiritual mission" was to synthesize science and religion. In 1879, he went to school in Vienna to study mathematics and science. There he met an influential Theosophist who drew him further into the sphere of the occult.

In 1886, Steiner was employed as a tutor to four boys, one of whom was an autistic ten-year-old. The boy's supposed "mental retardation" was attributed to hydrocephalus ("water on the brain"). In *Rudolf Steiner and Holistic Medicine* (1986), Francis X. King writes:

> Steiner came to the conclusion that there was nothing fundamentally wrong with the boy's mind; the real cause of the seeming mental retardation was that the undeveloped body was not working in harmony with the mind. . . . What was needed, decided Steiner, was to give the boy . . . "mental confidence." This, so he believed,

would result in [the boy's] mind and body working together in harmony, as nature . . . intended.

Steiner's confidence-boosting is alleged to have enabled the boy to become a medical doctor. But what surprised Steiner, says King, was that "the mental changes were accompanied by physical changes, the hydrocephaly steadily diminishing." Thus, Steiner concluded that "the state of the mind can be productive of physical changes in the human organism."

The Madame and the Mystic

Steiner became a superficial follower of Madame Blavatsky and a lecturer on mysticism. Blavatsky's death from influenza in 1891. By 1907, the Theosophical Society was led by Annie Besant, a social reformer, and Charles Webster Leadbeater, a pederastic former Anglican priest and so-called clairvoyant. Both preferred "Esoteric Christianity" to the "Esoteric Buddhism" that Blavatsky had propounded. In 1902, Steiner consulted with Besant in London. According to an article by macrobiotics proponent Ronald Kotzsch in the March 1984 *East West*, shortly after this meeting, Steiner addressed an audience in Berlin that included the elite of the German intellectual and academic communities and declared himself a Theosophist. He called for "a rejection of simple materialism as a basis for scientific research" and for the introduction of two concepts into the scientific enterprise: God and "the divine element in nature." Kotzsch describes Steiner's audience as stunned and dismayed. "For him to call himself a theosophist was to risk being associated with sleepwalkers, mediums, and spiritualist quacks," Kotzsch writes. "Steiner, in effect, had just come out of the 'spiritualist closet.'"

In 1902, Steiner also joined the Theosophical Society's German Section in Berlin and was installed as its general secretary, a position he held for a decade. But his academic training and philosophical leanings were at variance with Theosophy; he apparently had joined the German Section with the intention of taking control. Steiner was also leader of the society's German Esoteric Section and a member of the mystical Rosicrucian Brotherhood. As such, he emphasized "Christian Theosophy"—Western, rather than Eastern, mysticism. By 1907, largely because of his influence, the German Section was virtually independent in doctrine from the rest of the society.

On December 31, 1908, Besant proclaimed the imminent return of a messianic entity referred to as the "World Teacher" or "Christ." The following spring, on a beach near the society's headquarters in India,

Leadbeater met fourteen-year-old Jiddu Krishnamurti (1895-1986), referred to as "K" by his principal biographer. K's father, an impoverished widower, was employed as a clerk at the headquarters. Leadbeater is said to have marveled at the boy's "aura." By early 1910, Besant was certain that Lord Maitreya, a being greater than "the Masters," would become manifest through K's body. Thus, she and Leadbeater set about preparing K to be a "vehicle" or "conduit."

According to the Theosophical Society's founders, Maitreya had possessed Jesus Christ. In contrast, Steiner revered the life, death, and supposed resurrection of the "one and only" Jesus Christ as the most important developments in the history of the universe. Kotzsch writes:

> Blavatsky and Besant taught that all religions were more or less equal, providing different expressions of the same truth. Steiner allowed that all religions contained elements of the truth suitable for a particular time and place.
> But he insisted that the Christ event and the continued activity of the Christ in the world is unique.

Thus, Steiner considered the propaganda extolling K as the "new Christ-Incarnate" blasphemous and absurd, and was unable to abide the affair. In 1913, the German charter was returned to the Theosophical Society, and Steiner and the majority of the German Section formed the rival Anthroposophical Society in Dornach, Switzerland. This was devoted to acquiring wisdom primarily from man's "higher consciousness" rather than from alleged supernatural entities.

In 1929, K categorically rejected his demigod status and disowned organized religion across the board. On the day he renounced his messianic role, he told more than three thousand of his followers:

> A belief is purely an individual matter, and you cannot and must not organize it. If you do, it becomes dead, crystallized; it becomes a creed, a sect, a religion, to be imposed on others.
> This is what everyone throughout the world is attempting to do. . . . Truth cannot be brought down, rather the individual must make the effort to ascend to it. . . .
> The moment you follow someone you cease to follow Truth.

Patchwork Philosophy and the Quest for "Wholeness"

In contrast with theosophy, Anthroposophy means "man-wisdom." The word is now applied to Steiner's eclectic teachings, which encompass: (1) a system of body movements termed "eurythmy" or "eurhythmy" (so-called "visible speech," "visible song," or "sacred dance"); (2) a mode of education stressing art, drama, and "spiritual development," as embodied in the Anthroposophical Society's Waldorf Schools; (3) a bizarre theory of medicine; and (4) "biodynamic" agriculture, a peculiar type of "organic" farming. Steiner intended Anthroposophy to be an all-embracing science that would provide thoroughly satisfying answers in every branch of human endeavor. Yet, in *The Occult Establishment* (1976), James Webb writes:

> Steiner's ideas form less a "system" than an accumulation of sometimes apparently disconnected items. Thus, from Theosophy he took the ideas of *karma* and reincarnation; from his mystical studies . . . a personal "Rosicrucianism." He discovered an entirely new idiosyncratic and poetic interpretation of Christianity, and somehow contrived a seeming coherence with these teachings for theories of the social and artistic life of man. The underlying unity which he and his followers found in these elements of Anthroposophy lies in their source in Steiner's. . . . faculty of "clairvoyance."

Simply put, acceptance of Steiner's teachings rests ultimately on faith in his alleged extrasensory abilities. Steiner claimed to have access to the "Akashic Chronicle," or "Akashic Record," a supposed cosmic reservoir or library. The Chronicle is believed to preserve—in the form of impressions on the "astral plane"—every thought and action that has ever occurred in the material world since the beginning of the universe. These impressions are believed to be intelligible to psychics. Anthroposophy holds that the earth evolved through seven epochs and civilizations, with Lucifer and Ahriman (the Persian god of evil) forever opposing human progress. According to *The Universal Human: The Evolution of Individuality*, published in 1990 by the Anthroposophic Press, Steiner stated in 1909 that humanity's "clairvoyant consciousness" had declined since the "Atlantean catastrophe," but that this decline had enabled Christ to take human form. "However," he added, "we must not remain like this. We must ascend again into the spiritual world." Webb relates Steiner's belief that the (mythical) founder of the Rosicrucian Brotherhood (to which Steiner belonged) "sent his favorite pupil, Buddha, to Mars, where he . . . regenerated the planet as Christ had redeemed earth."

The Arkana Dictionary of New Perspectives (1989) defines eurythmy as "sound made manifest through gesture." King describes it as "a reflection in movement . . . of the great dance of creation, the activities of the Logos, the Word, of the opening verses of the Gospel according to Saint John. . . . an expression of the ultimate ground of all being." According to eurythmy, linguistic sounds have counterparts in postures and movements involving mainly the arms and hands. It has two derivatives: educational eurythmy and therapeutic, or curative, eurythmy. The latter form, says King, is used by Anthroposophical physicians against "a whole range of disorders" to "help restore a proper flow of the astral energies." "The curative power," explains Richard Grossinger in *Planet Medicine* (1987), "comes from the potentization of the alphabet, which translates the seed forms of these sounds into sequences which have meaning for the human personality and anatomy."

In the March 1984 issue of *East West* magazine, Ronald Kotzsch noted that the Anthroposophical Society had about twenty-five thousand members, with the greatest concentrations in Germany, Holland, and Switzerland, and about two thousand members in North America. He further stated that there were three hundred Waldorf Schools in twenty-one countries. A 1989–90 Rudolf Steiner College brochure stated that there were over four hundred such schools, about a hundred in the United States and Canada. A 1990 mailing from the Anthroposophical Society of America listed seventy in the United States. In 1989, according to Kotzsch, there were more than eighty of them in the United States, with about seven thousand students enrolled.

The unaccredited Rudolf Steiner College in Fair Oaks, California, was founded in 1976. It occupies thirteen acres and offers three full-time programs, an evening program, and an extension program in San Francisco. The three full-time programs include: an introductory program covering such topics as "Parsifal and the Quest for the Holy Grail"; a teacher education program; and an arts program, which, according to a brochure, "can lead to pedagogical or therapeutic application." All three programs cover eurythmy.

Kotzsch's 1984 article stated that there were about fifteen hundred biodynamic farms and gardening enterprises in the world. A 1990 directory published by the Anthroposophical Society of America states that its agricultural affiliate had certified twenty-one biodynamic farms in the United States and eleven "organic" farms in the United States and Mexico. "Biodynamics" is defined in the March/April 1992 *Real News* as the practice of working "with the energies that create and sustain life." According to "biodynamic" farmer Mack Mead, the main difference between "organic" and "biodynamic" farming lies in the treatment of the compost. In "biodynamic" farming, says Mead, most compost is "made from quite strong, healthy plants like nettles, valerian, and camomile, plants that are very strong and vital."

Illness as Blessing

Anthroposophical medicine is a combination of scientific medicine, homeopathy, and Anthroposophy. An article by Richard Leviton in the July 1988 *East West* claims that more than one thousand medical doctors "formally practice" Anthroposophical medicine and that another two thousand routinely prescribe Anthroposophical "remedies" from an extensive pharmacopoeia. According to Leviton, nearly fifty medical doctors were practicing Anthroposophical medicine in the United States by the late 1980s. He correctly describes the theory behind Anthroposophical medicine as "complex and detailed. . . . For those used to a conceptual perceptual framework, it can seem arcane, even baffling; it certainly requires hard study and long contemplation to master."

The fanciful physiology taught at the Waldorf School discussed in the beginning of this chapter lies at the foundation of Anthroposophical medicine, which endows the human organism with three systems: (1) a "neuro-sensorial" system, which supports sensation and thought; (2) a "metabolic-limb" (or "digestive-limb") system, which actualizes the will; and (3) a "rhythmic system" of circulation and respiration, which enables "feeling." Anthroposophical medicine postulates that the body has three "poles"—identified as "cool," "warm," and "balancing"—corresponding to these systems. The cool pole, localized in the head, represents the constantly dying cells of the nervous system—disintegration (catabolism). Anthroposophy holds that consciousness results from the decomposition of nerve cells, that it is a "death process." The warm pole, localized in the lower part of the organism, represents the active "metabolic cells"— integration (anabolism). The balancing pole, localized in the middle of the organism, supposedly acts as mediator between the cool and warm poles. Steiner believed that polar forces—anabolic ("warm") and catabolic ("cool")—function through the interplay of physical and spiritual (or "subtle") "bodies," as described below.

In *Anthroposophical Medicine* (1984), Victor Bott, M.D., writes that gravity, cosmic forces, and solar forces are designated "etheric" or "formative" forces by Anthroposophy. But, he adds:

> They must not be confused with the hypothetical vital force of which nineteenth-century science spoke. . . . Neither have they anything to do with the hypothetical ether of the physicists. These etheric or formative forces constitute for every living being a kind of second body, the *etheric body*, intimately united with the physical body which alone is accessible to our senses.

The objection that "etheric forces" are not visible, he asserts, is "no more valid than that which a color-blind person could make to the existence of colors." The "material support" or medium for these forces, writes Bott, is always water. During the growth of a plant, "the substances borrowed from the mineral world are . . . raised to the level of the vegetable kingdom." Thus, Anthroposophists believe that plants have an "etheric body" in addition to the physical body of "mineral-organisms." Animals are thought to have, in addition, an "astral body" or "soul body." Humans are thought to possess a physical body, an etheric body, an astral body, and—unlike minerals, plants, and animals—a phase referred to as the ego, ego-consciousness, ego-organization, or human spirit. The ego is supposedly "born" at age twenty-one. The plant-related etheric body is supposedly born at age seven and composed of formative, reparative forces. The animal-related astral body is born at age fourteen. Supposedly home to emotions, it is said to consume the plant-related formative forces, thus making consciousness possible. Steiner maintained that health is dependent upon the harmonious interaction of the physical, etheric, and astral bodies with one another and with the ego.

Anthroposophists view illness as imbalance or disharmony—hyperactivity of the warm or cool poles—and regard it as an opportunity to achieve "wholeness." Toward this end, Steiner advocated the use of animal, mineral, and plant substances. Anthroposophical remedies are supposed to restore balance either by strengthening the therapeutic, plant-related "etheric body" or by moderating the animalistic "astral body."

According to a 1990 issue of the *ANTHA Newsletter*, published by the Anthroposophical Therapy and Hygiene Association, in Spring Valley, New York, "Anthroposophically-extended" medicine is similar overall to homeopathy, but differs in both the preparation of remedies and the method by which they are selected. In Anthroposophy, the source of the medicinal substance is important, because different sources—as of silica or calcium—"point to different creative processes." Each mineral substance—quartz, onyx, oyster shell, coral, and marble, for example—supposedly carries different healing forces. Furthermore, both the time of day and "planet constellations" are considered in the preparation of remedies. They are not prepared between noon and 3:00 P.M.—the time of day considered "the least alive." The aim of the Anthroposophical physician is not to terminate the disease process, but to regulate it to facilitate the patient's attainment of "wholeness."

Leviton quotes an Anthroposophical physician practicing in a Steiner-based elderly care facility in Spring Valley, New York: "Illness can be considered a friend, a teacher, a blessing in disguise. It teaches a person what needs to be done in consciousness. . . . An illness is wasted if a person is not transformed by it." In the same article, another Anthroposophical physician contends that childhood immunizations are "damaging" because they increase the incidence of degenerative disease in later life. Leviton also quotes Dr. Otto Wolff, a leading exponent of Anthroposophical medicine and editor of the three-volume *Anthroposophical Approach to Medicine*. Wolff defines healing as "bringing oneself into harmony with the divine creative force." According to him, "One who does not nurture spiritual life is bound eventually to become ill"; yet illness is the path to "the restitution of the divine archetype of humanity."

Leviton cites several Anthroposophical remedies, including: (1) *Formica*, derived from red ants, "to help bring dead matter back into the life cycle"; (2) *Magnesium phosphoricum*, "to introduce more light"; (3) a copper preparation "for the kidneys"; and (4) meteoric iron "for the pancreas." In addition to unscientific "remedies" and curative eurythmy, the Anthroposophical physician may prescribe color therapy, meditation, music, prayer, and social service projects. Another remedy associated with Anthroposophy is iscador (also called *Viscum album*), a mistletoe preparation that Steiner first proposed for treating cancer in 1920. The American Cancer Society considers iscador an "unproven remedy" and has strongly advised against its use.

In *Man and World in the Light of Anthroposophy* (1989), Stewart C. Easton states that "in anthroposophical medical practice it is virtually impossible to use a 'book of rules'. . . . A developed insight, through which at least the *workings* of unseen forces can be recognized, is absolutely essential." And Kotzsch writes:

> This strong religious and Christian orientation is not always apparent in the practical activities of the anthroposophical movement. Yet each [activity] in its own way seeks to encourage and aid this evolution to a selfless love of God, the divine beings, nature, and our fellow humans. Biodynamic farming produces foodstuffs which will nourish the spirit as well as the body. Anthroposophical medicine treats the social and spiritual dimension of the patient, not only the physical.

Since 1931, Anthroposophical remedies have been marketed in the United States through the Weleda Corporation, now located in Spring Valley, New York. The company also sells books on Anthroposophy by Steiner and by other authors.

A "Reality-Based" Nutritional "Hygiene"?

Although nutrition and dietetics are a significant feature of Anthroposophy, its philosophy in this regard is not easily extracted. Steiner devoted at least two or three lectures to nutrition, but never gave a course on the subject. Easton writes: "Steiner did not declare himself in favor of certain diets, and . . . he was careful to comment that . . . he was not *advocating* any particular dietary practice."

Today, the leading exponent of Anthroposophical nutrition seems to be Gerhard Schmidt. Originally published in 1975 in German, his *Dynamics of Nutrition* (1980) is subtitled: *The Impulse of Rudolf Steiner's Spiritual Science for a New Nutritional Hygiene*. Schmidt writes: "As fragmentary as it may appear in isolation, Rudolf Steiner developed a new and reality-based conception of the field of nutrition." He admits that, because he "tried to approach Rudolf Steiner's method of working," his book lacks a systematic presentation.

According to Schmidt, nutrition "serves to stimulate and unfold the health-giving forces of the etheric body." It is thus "active against the death forces and has . . . the task of preventing disease." He advises that if disease gains the upper hand in any way, medication must be supplemented with a special diet to stimulate the innately health-promoting etheric body. But the diet should not jeopardize the astral or "soul body." The latter is described as "the carrier of disease processes," yet necessary for the functioning of the ego-consciousness by virtue of these selfsame processes. Recall that Anthroposophists believe consciousness is the result of cellular decomposition. In Schmidt's words: "Through the destruction of substance, space is created for the development of thought life." In *Fundamentals of Therapy*, completed only three days before his death, Steiner and clinician Dr. Ita Wegman stated: "It is only because the human organism is decaying . . . that the soul and spirit can have the human organism as their basis."

Schmidt defines healing as having "the possibility to bring about activities in the etheric body which oppose the disease-provoking effects of the astral body." He explains:

> We can only maintain ourselves against the destructive effect of nature if we are able to provide sufficient resistance against it. Food gives us the stimulation, the means, to unfold these [resisting] forces within ourselves. Thus we do not take in the substance and forces of nature in order to utilize them directly, but rather to

create through them the forces which counter the destructive forces of nature.... It is through nutrition that we must bring about this transformation in the right way.

The "life forces" of plants, according to Schmidt, oppose the destructive forces of nature and are thus healthful. "A living plant," he says, "is filled with forces that take its substance into spheres which are cosmic rather than earthly." Man is "involved with" the "etheric formative forces of the plants when he eats plant foods.... [which] continue to be active in the plant even when it has been picked." However, the plant "must lose its life"—undergo "de-vitalization"—before man's etheric and astral bodies can assimilate it. Similarly, "animal food must... be divested of its typical animalistic character." Schmidt states that if "the forces needed to overcome foods from plants and animals" are "not awakened," underutilized, or "allowed to atrophy through disease," they will "recoil back into the organism"; "their effect on man is then very tiring and disturbing." Animal foods, he says, are easily "overcome" or "humanized" by man. But a "doubled effort" is supposedly needed to "overcome" plant foods; they are thought to be more healthful in consequence of this greater capacity for stimulation. Uncooked food is considered therapeutic for the same reason: In the booklet *Cancer and Nutrition,* published by the Anthroposophical Press in 1986, Schmidt conveys that although cooked food "is a kind of basis for human nutrition," uncooked foods need "stronger forces to be overcome" and thus are particularly recommended in cases of pathological skin conditions and of tumors."

In *The Essentials of Nutrition* (1987), his sequel to *The Dynamics of Nutrition,* Schmidt calls sauerkraut "a special dietary food" and indicates that if oxalic acid does not "develop" in the human digestive tract, life cannot be sustained. Oxalic acid is both a byproduct of human metabolism and a food constituent—present, for example, in cocoa and spinach. As a food constituent, it interferes with the absorption of calcium, magnesium, and iron.

Anthroposophy advocates a largely lactovegetarian, or semivegetarian, diet with an emphasis on "biodynamically grown" foodstuffs. Schmidt expresses Steiner's teaching that during the so-called Lemurian epoch "mother's milk came to man as food from his surrounding atmosphere." He says today's milk is "an after-image of the original cosmic nutrition.... the bridge between cosmic and earthly nutrition." In a 1924 lecture, Steiner said:

There are people who simply cannot live if they don't have meat. A person must consider carefully whether he really will be able to get on without it. . . . If, however, one does become a vegetarian, he feels stronger—because he is no longer obliged to deposit alien fat in his body; he makes his own fat.

The Bottom Line

It is a formidable task to decipher or even to summarize Anthroposophy's gibberish. I have given the latter my best shot. Apparently, some people take comfort in Anthroposophy's bizarre spiritism. Its position on diet appears physically innocuous. Its hostility toward scientific health care is not.

9

Gerson Therapy: Method or Madness?

"Medical Fact"?

Gerson therapy is a "nutritional" approach that is also referred to as Gerson treatment, the Gerson dietary regime, and the Gerson method. A 1992 Gerson Institute flyer characterizes it as:

> A state of the art, contemporary, wholistic and natural treatment which assists the body's own healing mechanism. The clinical results it produces still frequently stretch the imaginations of capable scientists and physicians because science does not yet know how it works. The effects of nutrition and metabolism on immunity are not yet understood, but the ability of the Gerson Therapy to improve, extend survival, and cure chronic and advanced diseases is medical fact.

Max Gerson: Genius or Quack?

Born in Wongrowitz, Germany, Max B. Gerson, M.D. (1881–1959), originated the first so-called metabolic therapy—alleged to cure by "detoxification." He attended the universities of Breslau, Wuerzburg, Berlin, and Freiburg, and studied under Professor Ottfried Foerster, a renowned neurosurgeon. In medical school, Gerson suffered from severe migraines for which he was told there was no remedy. Undaunted, he sought relief by adjusting his diet, using apples as the basis for adding other foods. In the process, he allegedly found that his headaches could be "controlled" by a "natural foods" diet emphasizing fresh fruits and vegetables and excluding fats, salt, and pickled and smoked foods.

Gerson graduated from medical school in Freiburg in 1906. Under the aegis of Ferdinand Sauerbruch, a famous thoracic surgeon and authority on tuberculosis, Gerson became director of the tuberculosis department of the Munich University Hospital. Encouraged by his personal experience, Gerson made his "migraine diet" part of his medical practice. One of his patients who had been following the diet for a few weeks on Gerson's instructions not only claimed it had relieved his migraines, but insisted it had cured him of tuberculosis of the skin (lupus vulgaris), considered incurable at the time. Lab tests allegedly supported the patient's latter claim, and Gerson began putting tuberculosis patients on his diet.

During the mid-1920s, Gerson practiced medicine in Bielefeld, Germany, specializing in diseases of the nervous system, yet treating tuberculosis patients with diet. The medical community objected to his venturing outside of his area of specialization and attempted to revoke his license. Gerson responded by changing his shingle from one reading "Internal and Nervous Diseases" to one reading "General Practitioner," and began prescribing his diet for other diseases, including meningitis, diabetes, arteriosclerosis, arthritis, all other forms of tuberculosis, and, in 1928, cancer. His original "anticancer" diet consisted of fresh vegetables and fruits (many raw) and freshly prepared juices, with gradual addition of buttermilk, cottage cheese, yogurt, and raw egg yolks. A multimineral supplement and frequent enemas were given along with the diet. In subsequent years, fresh "green leaf juice," fresh raw calf's liver juice, injections of raw liver extract, desiccated thyroid gland, potassium supplements, and coffee enemas were added.

Gerson lectured in the principal cities of Europe until 1933, when the prewar political climate prompted him to escape from Nazi Germany. He was well into his fifties when he emigrated to the United States in 1936. In 1938 he passed the state board examination in New York State, was granted a license to practice medicine, and resumed prescribing his regimen to private patients. Meanwhile, his parents and seven siblings were murdered in concentration camps.

"No Actual Cure"

In 1945, the *Review of Gastroenterology* published a report of Gerson's findings, entitled "Dietary Considerations in Malignant Neoplastic Diseases." The article described his therapy in detail and included ten case-history abstracts. The Gerson treatment comprised four dietary stages plus supplements of calcium, vitamin A, vitamin D_2 (a synthetic form that rarely occurs in nature), niacin, powdered desiccated bile from young animals, defatted liver powder, and injectable crude liver extract.

In the report, Gerson described the "cancer version" of his diet, or Modified Gerson Diet, as: (1) salt-free, (2) fat-free ("all vegetables or foods containing fats, fatty acids or lecithin are excluded"), (3) low in animal proteins, (4) high in minerals of what he called the "K-group" (potassium and the other predominant intracellular ions—phosphate and magnesium), (5) high in complex carbohydrates, (6) abundant in fluid, (7) rich in vitamins, and (8) "rich in some liver substances and enzymes." Gerson's "forbidden food" list included: (1) salt, other sodium com-pounds, and most spices; (2) coffee, tea, cocoa, and alcoholic beverages; (3) all canned, preserved, and bottled foods; (4) white flour and white sugar (brown sugar and molasses were allowed); (5) chocolate and candies in general, cakes, and ice cream (apple pie made with rye flour and raisins was allowed after four weeks of therapy); (6) all animal and vegetable fats; (7) nuts; (8) pineapples, berries, pomegranates, and a type of pear; and (9) mushrooms.

The case history abstracts are not very detailed and do not indicate which components of the Gerson treatment were utilized. Three abstracts do not specify when the treatment began, but it apparently began less than three years before publication of the article in all ten cases, less than two years in seven cases, and less than a year in two cases. To be meaningful, cancer survival statistics usually require longer follow-up periods. In addition, four of the patients cited had undergone both cancer surgery and radiation therapy before adopting Gerson's treatment, and the remaining patients had undergone either surgery or radiotherapy. At the outset of his summary, Gerson himself conceded: "In all of these patients . . . no actual cure has occurred."

In 1947, the National Cancer Institute reviewed ten cases selected by Gerson and was left unconvinced. That same year, a committee appointed by the New York County Medical Society reviewed the records of eighty-six cancer patients, examined ten patients, and found no scientific evidence of benefit.

In 1949, *Experimental Medicine and Surgery* published a report in which Gerson described five cases of malignant tumors and one of "borderline malignancy." Three of the patients had undergone both cancer surgery and radiotherapy prior to Gerson's intervention, and one had undergone extensive surgery. None had followed the regimen for more than about four years, and one had followed it for less than two years. Gerson himself concluded that it was "too early to make any definite statement" about the value of his regimen.

From 1946 to 1950, Gerson treated patients at the Gotham Hospital in New York City. He also operated inpatient treatment facilities in New York State for more than a decade, from 1948 until the year of his death. However, his malpractice insurance was discontinued in 1953. In 1956, during a question-and-answer session following a lecture he delivered in Escondido, California, Gerson confessed that he had "damaged" patients with vitamins A, E, and B_6, declared that vitamin D "is picked up by the cancer cells immediately," stated that calcium administration could cause cancer, and advised against using calcium, magnesium, and other minerals.

In 1957, a special subcommittee of the New York County Medical Society was appointed to review the Gerson method. The subcommittee concluded:

> The nine cases that were officially reported were found to indicate that Dr. Gerson demonstrated a lack of understanding of the natural history of [cancer]. His presentation of cases left much to be desired in the way of either proof that some patients actually had [cancer] at the time they were treated or that actual cure or arrest of the malignant process, if present, had resulted from his treatment. He showed no case in which it could be demonstrated that a cure of [cancer] had been obtained by his treatment.

In 1958, after a lengthy investigation, the Society voted to suspend Gerson's membership.

The first edition of Gerson's *A Cancer Therapy: Results of Fifty Cases* was published shortly after his death in 1959. Subtitled *The Cure of Advanced Cancer by Diet Therapy*, the book has undergone four subsequent editions and remains in print. In it Gerson spoke of "the laws of nature," "life activators," "life stimulating substances," "*vital* processes," "the healing power," the "soul," and "Eternal Life." He referred to the nervous system as our "spiritual organ." He advocated consumption of "organically grown" fruits and vegetables, especially to treat cancer, citing that "life begets life." He pointed out a need for "real housewives, not eager to save kitchen time," and acknowledged that "the practice of the treatment is a difficult task" requiring "somebody's help all day long." Gerson indicted science and technology as mainly responsible for "evil" and stated that it was "necessary . . . to bring medical doctrine back nearer to nature."

He described cancer as due ultimately not to carcinogens but to a cumulative "poisoning" of the digestive organs, chiefly the liver, by foodstuffs he alleged to be deficient in the so-called K-group. This deficiency, he claimed, was the result of modern agricultural practices such as artificial fertilization.

Because of Politics?

The Gerson Institute in Bonita, California, functions as an information and referral service for Gerson therapy and publishes a newsletter titled *Healing*, which features interviews with "healed" patients and "alternative" medicine proponents. The Institute was founded in 1977 by Gerson's daughter, Charlotte, and former aerospace engineer Norman Fritz as a non-profit, member-supported educational organization. Membership, which costs $15 or more annually, includes a subscription to the newsletter.

Ms. Gerson (often referred to as Charlotte Gerson Strauss), who serves as Institute president, was born in post-World War I Germany. She left with her family in 1933 and continued her education in Austria, France, and England, completing her studies in the United States. She attended her father's lectures, assisted in translating his writings into English, and helped manage his clinics. In recent years she has lectured throughout the United States and in Canada and Austria, and has appeared on many talk shows. She maintains that "all chronic diseases are deficiency diseases."

The Gerson Therapy Center of Mexico at La Gloria, about six miles south of Tijuana, opened in 1977, but was shut down in 1985 after an extensive fire. After temporarily operating at a motel in Tijuana one mile from the U.S. border, it reopened as Hospital de Baja California, a for-profit facility described in an Institute flyer as "a modern day sanatorium." In July 1991, it was renamed Centro Hospitalario Internacional del Pacifico, S.A. (CHIPSA), which *Healing* describes as "the first accredited hospital in the Western Hemisphere dedicated to the care of people with a wide range of diseases and using the Gerson Therapy as primary treatment."

The "full intensive" Gerson therapy, as described in a 1992 Gerson Institute flyer, consists of: (1) thirteen glasses a day of raw juices prepared hourly from fresh, "organically grown" fruits and vegetables; (2) three full vegetarian meals, freshly prepared from "organically grown" foodstuffs; (3) multiple enemas of coffee and/or chamomile tea; and (4) medications including a potassium compound, thyroid hormone, Lugol's solution (a strong iodine medication), injectable crude liver extract with vitamin B_{12}, pancreatic enzymes, and castor oil. Three "adjuvant treatments" are specified in the 1992 flyer: ozone, hydrotherapy, and an intravenous infusion of "GKI"—a solution of glucose, potassium, and insulin. The 1991 flyer, however, lists a total of six "adjuvant treatments," including hydrogen peroxide, "live cell therapy," and packs of castor oil and/or clay. The castor oil packs are prepared and used as recommended by Edgar Cayce. The fruit and vegetable "juices" are actually composed of crushed pulp.

The 1992 flyer claims that Gerson therapy can cure allergies, angina, arterial inflammation, arthritis, asthma, atherosclerosis, bronchitis, advanced cancer, cirrhosis, colitis, diabetes, eczema, edema, "chronic" Epstein-Barr virus, chronic hepatitis, hypertension, migraines, multiple sclerosis, psoriasis, lupus, and tuberculosis. The suggested length of stay is three to six weeks, with a deposit of at least $3,900 (cash or traveler's checks) required prior to each week of treatment. The basic daily charge is $495 plus 10 percent tax. Prospective patients are encouraged to bring a companion, at an additional cost of $40 per day plus tax. A 1992 Gerson Institute mailing states:

> The Gerson Therapy offers patients with cancer, or other so-called 'incurable' diseases, a good chance of winning if they follow the therapy diligently. If the therapy principles are applied as a way of life, almost all 'incurable' diseases are prevented. A long and high-quality life is the result. Then heart disease, strokes, cancer, diabetes, arthritis, and the other diseases of civilization that kill and cripple us will not occur.

In September 1992, I received a postcard announcing that CBS News would give Gerson therapy "several minutes of favorable nationwide exposure." The notice even proffered videotapes at $7.00 apiece. However, when I phoned the Institute, I was told that the segment had been canceled "because of politics."

The President and the Prophet

In 1988, Charlotte Gerson was interviewed for more than two and a half hours on cable television by Elizabeth Clare Prophet, president and co-founder of the Church Universal and Triumphant, and author of *The Lost Years of Jesus*. Prophet purports to be a messenger for the "Ascended Masters." (As noted in Chapter 8, the original "Masters" were invented by Madame H.P. Blavatsky, co-founder of the Theosophical Society.) The

Fall 1991 issue of *Free Inquiry* reported that during 1989 and 1990 about four thousand of her church members responded to her prediction of imminent nuclear holocaust by selling their homes, relocating to her headquarters in Montana, and buying bomb shelters from the church at prices as high as $12,000.

In the interview, Ms. Gerson said that her father had been called a "fraud," a "rip-off," and a "cruel hoax, giving cancer patients false hope ... and ripping them off for huge sums." Prophet responded: "If they cannot find anything to expose you on, then they [fabricate] the lie out of the whole cloth. And this has been going on a long time against the true revolutionaries."

The therapy's basis, Gerson said, "is detoxifying the body and rebuilding it. And that's easy to say, but it requires a great deal of work." She described enzymes as "activators" and said that "toxins" or "poisons" were "enzyme inhibitors." She asserted:

We get a lot of poisons nowadays, in the air, in the water, in the soil, in our plants, in the food, in the processed foods, in dyes and emulsifiers, and in ... chemicals of all sorts that are additives to food. And they do damage in the human body. And being chemicals, and being toxins, they inhibit enzymes. And if you inhibit enzymes, you cannot activate the body. So the first thing you have to do is get rid of these toxins.

Her father, she said, had accomplished this with fresh juices and coffee enemas. Fresh juices, she explained, help "to flush out and wash out the system." She said that a post-World War I study, in which caffeine was introduced into the rectum of animals, had shown that "the caffeine does proceed ... into the liver area, and it opens the liver and bile ducts and allows for these toxins that are blocking the body to be released and eliminated through the liver and bile ducts."

Prophet shortly announced: "Whoever hears this information may, to his benefit or detriment, experiment with some of the things we are saying." But she emphasized that Gerson therapy is "a total program ... not the treatment of disease," but "treatment of the body and especially the restoration of the immune system." When she requested specifics on the coffee enemas, Gerson obliged: Three rounded tablespoons of coffee are added to a quart of boiling water. The coffee should boil for two to three minutes, then simmer for about twenty minutes. After simmering, the coffee is strained, and four to five tablespoons of castor oil and two to three drops of an emulsifier such as Castile or *Ivory* soap are added. The enema is given at body temperature, should be held for twelve to fifteen minutes, and should be repeated every four hours. In an interview in the April 1991 issue of Swanson Health Products' *Health Shopper*, she said that coffee enemas "stimulate the discharge of accumulated toxins from the liver-bile system" and attributed this alleged effect to caffeine.

To Prophet and her audience, Charlotte Gerson said: "We have to be very careful here." Caffeine alone, she cautioned, won't do the trick: "Coffee beans are extremely high in potassium. The potassium is important for the intestinal tract because without potassium, there's cramping and spasming." Moreover, she warned that "overusing" coffee enemas is "perfectly possible if, for instance, you use it according to the book [*A Cancer Therapy*]—say, every four hours—but you don't use the juices." Under these circumstances, she said, "you get an electrolyte imbalance: you wash out too many minerals without restoring them."

However, she added: "The time comes, sometimes, when patients get healing reactions—flare-ups—when the body really lets go, and they feel very sloppy; they can feel nausea. . . . At those times, they can't drink all that much juice; they sometimes vomit."

Ms. Gerson enumerated the juices used in Gerson therapy: (1) orange juice; (2) "green juice," made from such salad vegetables as green peppers, chard, and red cabbage, and including one whole apple per glass; (3) carrot and apple juice; and (4) liver juice. She said it is very important to add an apple to the green juice "because it gives the pectin to the intestinal tract so that the body can handle all these somewhat harsh raw vegetables and juices."

Later she said: "We always have to remember that the Gerson therapy is not designed as a treatment for cancer." But she thereupon described the case of a fifty-one-year-old fireman with prostate cancer, painful kidney stones, three herniated disks, sciatica, and high blood pressure, who had lost "about 50 percent of his muscle mass from atrophy." Ms. Gerson credited the Gerson therapy not only with allegedly clearing his prostate of cancer, but for dissolving his kidney stones, restoring his disks and muscle mass, relieving his sciatica, and lowering his blood pressure. Prophet interpreted that the patient had been "delivered in a single day," and designated *A Cancer Therapy* "the Bible." She later stated: "We do not treat disease. We make no claims for the cure of disease. We make claims for the restoration of the body by itself—when you give it the right things."

"When the body is given the right nutrients, is given help in detoxifying," Gerson agreed, "it will heal itself." Prophet emphasized: "We can't cure cancer. Only our bodies can cure the cancer if we will just cooperate."

"Funny Things" Can Happen

Ms. Gerson branded as poison "any sodium that's added to what is naturally contained in the foods we eat." Potassium, on the other hand, was a remedy she said her father had administered "in large amounts" to terminally ill cancer patients with above-normal serum concentrations of potassium. She said her father had recommended the gluconate, acetate, and phosphate forms of potassium—but not potassium chloride, "which can be dangerous." However, she added that potassium pills don't always replenish the cells, and that for best results the potassium must be in a "live" form, such as in cherries, apricots, peaches, and plums.

She further stressed the alleged safety of the potassium compound used at the Gerson Therapy Center. "Some funny things happen," she said. Then she related the story of a patient who had returned home from the center with a three-month supply of the potassium compound, which she had been instructed to dissolve in one quart of water. The label on the bottle bore the same instructions. The patient phoned Ms. Gerson to complain that she had run out of the potassium compound too soon. "So she had taken," Gerson explained, "like a ten-times overdose of an already heroic dose of potassium—and nothing happened. . . . This has happened several times. No problem." She stated that, unlike potassium chloride, the Gerson potassium compound does not cause heart problems or other damage.

In addition to giving potassium by mouth, the Gerson Therapy Center provides potassium by injection into a vein. According to Ms. Gerson, this method—which she referred to as "polarizing treatment"—is reserved for "certain patients with a special need." The intravenous solution used at the center also contains glucose and insulin. Gerson gave her interpretation of a French physician's rationale for combining the three substances:

You got to get the potassium right into the fluid systems. . . . But it takes more than potassium: it takes the energy to force it into the cells, to let the sodium out and force the potassium into the cells. And in order to get that energy . . . you need a little glucose . . . and a little insulin—the insulin and glucose producing the energy, plus the potassium to restore the cell systems.

"It's ingenious, isn't it?" said Prophet.

When Gerson declared that patients at the center "get real, honest nutrition," Prophet responded: "I think some people here wish they had something wrong with them so they could come to your clinic—just some little thing." "You'd be surprised," Gerson told her. "A lot of people come just to detoxify . . . just to learn what to do and just to prevent disease. . . .

And it's wise. It's much easier to prevent than to cure." To these motivations Prophet added "rejuvenation." But Gerson later stated that about 70 percent of persons admitted to the Gerson Therapy Center are cancer patients. "The first signal of cancer," she declared, "very often is tiredness." Other signs to watch for, she stated, include depression and a "weakened and damaged" liver.

"If you're in generally pretty fair health," said Gerson, "you're likely to get a healing reaction"—including nausea, vomiting, and fever—"in two or three days. If you're really very seriously ill, it may take five or seven days. And then, we have seen patients whose healing reaction only lasts a couple of hours—they're not able to heal more than that much. Then we have seen others that are not really that ill, where the healing reaction can last three days. And they're miserable, but they are better off, because their body is getting rid of the toxins, getting rid of the waste and the accumulated damage. Their bodies are responding." Gerson concluded:

Once [people] realize that everything—that whether it's cancer or AIDS, or whether it's drug addiction or whether it's diabetes—that everything is really basically the same, and that it can all be prevented and/or handled and healed, you know that even then, a very large percentage of the people don't want to be bothered. But those who do, I think, are going to have to be there, and will have to be the leaders, because the others will be eliminated by nature; they will die.

"You've Got to Please Believe"

In May 1991, I attended a lecture given by Charlotte Gerson at a public school in Jamaica, New York. During the lecture, she asserted:

- "All drugs—no matter what reason they're given—all drugs are eventually liver toxic." (Yet she later stated that therapy at the center includes intramuscular injections of vitamin B_{12} and coffee enemas, and may include laetrile. In the Prophet interview, she herself had described coffee as a "drug.")

- Gerson therapy cures atherosclerosis, cancer, cardiac arrhythmias, diabetes mellitus, migraines, multiple sclerosis, "stroke problems," and tuberculosis, and normalizes high blood pressure.

- "Salt is a toxin, a poison."

- "You can't get fat unless you eat the wrong foods."

- Enzyme supplements "help the body digest and break down the tumor tissue."

- "Part of the problem of the cancer patient is that he's not able to digest animal fats and protein. They're not broken down to the end product [because] the enzyme systems are blocked. And when they're not digested to the end product, your cell systems aren't getting these nutrients. But the tumor tissue thrives on it, grabs all it can. And the fats and proteins you eat feed the tumor and starve your body."

- "The body needs its nutrients in their live, active form."

- "The human body is not designed for meat eating. We don't have the teeth of meat-eating animals." (She added: "Meat-eating is just totally wrong.")

- "Milk is a killer. . . . milk, cheese, fish, chicken, eggs, all of those things."

- "Cucumbers . . . just simply do not agree with [dietary] juices. Cucumbers and juices lie in the stomach like lead, and you can't digest them."

- "When the doctors tell you you have an incurable disease, always remember to add in the back of your mind: 'Yes, incurable by his methods.'"

Scientific treatment facilities and state health departments maintain tumor registries to systematically keep track of cancer patients through questionnaires sent to attending physicians at regular intervals. During the question-and-answer period I asked whether the Institute had a follow-up program. Sounding somewhat irritated, she replied:

We do not do that. The hospital people do. See, what the people who have been at the hospital—they're usually followed up by the doctors there, not so much by us. So we [have] had more, sort of haphazard, accidental information on the people who are still well. We don't always have the opportunity to follow up. When you write to people and ask them to answer questions, you get perhaps between 10 and 25 percent responses. You know, it's very difficult to get people to answer questionnaires and so on. We've got some of that. But we're not doctors, okay? Many patients we hear [from or about] accidentally . . . . And we hear, you know, from relatives and friends and neighbors and—and former Dr. Gerson patients.

Gerson said that patients at the Gerson Therapy Center undergo treatment with training for "maybe four weeks sometimes" and then go home. She added:

> But they have to do this [regimen] for two years. How do we know what they do at home? Many admit to cheating. Some don't know if they do something wrong. They don't know if they're in a toxic environment, or [if] the neighbor sprays and paints or something like that.... All kinds of things can happen. So basically we don't really want to do statistics—for other reasons, too: If we do statistics, we're gonna [have] the orthodox people come and say, "Hey, wait a minute—25 percent [of patients recovered]? We get 30 percent" . . . So it doesn't make sense for us to do statistics.

Another attendee inquired: "Is there any way . . . for a single person to follow the intensive therapy? Is it practically possible?" Gerson responded: "For a single person who is also ill, and who also has to make a living, it's almost impossible. You need to have help. You need to hire a helper." She also assured us that "there's a reason for everything" in the Gerson regimen. "If there was an explanation for each item that's forbidden, and for each item how to and why to and why not, the book [*A Cancer Therapy*] would be ten thousand pages. Okay? So you've got to please believe that there are reasons for each of these do's and don'ts."

Therapy or Penance?

In 1980 the *Journal of the American Medical Association* published a report on patients who had died as a result of electrolyte imbalance caused by coffee enemas. The first patient took ten or twelve coffee enemas one night and continued at a rate of one per hour in an attempt to relieve pain caused by gallstones. The second patient, who had metastatic breast cancer, began taking coffee enemas four times daily for two weeks at the Gerson Clinic and continued this routine after she returned home. The American Cancer Society's 1989 position paper warns against the use of the Gerson method for any medical condition.

Patients undergoing "detoxification" through Gerson therapy are likely to experience such symptoms as headache, fever, nausea, and intestinal spasms. Yet they may be told that such reactions signify the elimination of toxins from the body (the equivalent of what macrobiotic enthusiasts call "discharging"). In an interview in a late 1990 issue of *Healing*, a Gerson patient diagnosed with colorectal cancer described the "terrible time" he had taking coffee enemas through a colostomy: "It gave me the dry heaves. I was emotionally spent. It was something I couldn't deal with. I never realized how toxic I was."

More than a dozen Gerson patients have arrived comatose at San Diego hospitals as a result of electrolyte imbalances. According to the February 1986 issue of *Nutrition Forum*, a doctor with the San Diego Department of Health stated that within the previous six years, at least thirteen patients reportedly treated at the La Gloria center had been admitted to hospitals in the San Diego area with *Campylobacter* sepsis. Health officials considered raw calf's liver the likeliest source of the infection. In a 1990 issue of *Healing*, editor and Gerson Institute executive director Gar Hildenbrand writes that in October 1989 the Gerson Therapy Center stopped using raw calf's liver juice. He acknowledges that this decision "was based on multiple outbreaks of *Campylobacter gastroenteritis* at Hospital de Baja California in which symptoms were noted in up to 50% of hospitalized patients during one incident. Campylobacter was cultured from stool samples of affected patients. Veal liver was found to be the source of bacteria."

The *Nutrition Forum* article also describes a case reported by William T. Jarvis, Ph.D., wherein a 24-year-old osteopathic student with testicular cancer underwent surgery but refused chemotherapy because of his religious beliefs. Instead, he undertook Gerson therapy and other unproven methods consistent with his notion of "God's remedies." Although with proper treatment he would have had a 90 percent chance of surviving for five years, he died at the age of twenty-six. The same issue cites the case of a young woman who underwent conventional therapy but feared a recurrence. Her doctor performed a physical examination and discovered no evidence of cancer. Unconvinced, she turned to La Gloria, where she was told she had breast cancer. Following Gerson therapy for several weeks, however, made her so miserable she abandoned it and returned home—whereupon her doctor reassured her that no cancer was present.

Perhaps the most noteworthy study of Gerson therapy was reported in *Options: The Alternative Cancer Therapy Book* (1993), by Richard Walters. The study was done by Steve Austin, a naturopath who teaches nutrition at a chiropractic college. In 1983, he visited the Gerson Clinic and asked about thirty cancer patients to permit him to follow their progress. He was able to track twenty-one of them over a five-year period (or until death) through annual letters or phone calls. At the five-year mark, only one was still alive; the rest had succumbed to their cancer. The study is remarkable because Austin was favorably predisposed toward Gerson therapy. He and two colleagues also tracked twenty-two cancer patients who had received "metabolic therapy" (laetrile plus nutritional treatment) at the Mexican facility run by the Contreras family. In the December 1991 *Townsend Letter for Doctors*, a publication for "alternative" practitioners, they reported that all had died of their cancer within two years.

In 1991, *The New England Journal of Medicine* published the report of a study comparing the survival time and quality of life of seventy-eight terminal cancer patients undergoing "alternative" treatment at the Livingston-Wheeler Medical Clinic in San Diego with matched controls treated conventionally. The authors had hypothesized that the Livingston-Wheeler patients would experience a better quality of life because of the self-care components of the program and the absence of chemotherapy side effects. As expected, they found no difference in survival time, but contrary to their expectations, they found that the Livingston-Wheeler patients had a significantly lower quality of life. Since Gerson therapy is far more arduous, I suspect that its followers would do even more poorly.

The negative results found among patients who underwent Gerson therapy should come as no surprise, because the theories on which it is based are not valid. Saul Green, Ph.D., a former Sloan-Kettering researcher, has examined six theories upon which the Gerson approach is founded. In the December 9, 1992 *Journal of the American Medical Association*, he concludes:

> The poisons in processed foods that proponents of the Gerson therapy say cause cancer have never been identified. Frequent coffee enemas have never been shown to mobilize and remove poisons from the liver and the intestines of cancer patients. There is no evidence that "poisoned" oxidative enzymes in the liver and intestine are related to the onset of cancer. Enzymes in animal and vegetable foods cannot reach or replace enzymes in vital organs.... Of all the dietary regimens suggested as a treatment for cancer, none have ever been found to be more effective than the placebos that were used as controls.

The Bottom Line

The Gerson approach is based on "detoxification" and other simplistic notions that may sound scientific to laypersons. It is very costly and time-consuming. Its promoters—though claiming high cure rates—have never collected meaningful follow-up data on their patients. Case reviews by others indicated that Gerson therapy had no value whatsoever, and some cases of serious direct harm have been reported. But hope springs eternal in the hearts and pocketbooks of desperate patients and their families.

10

The Matol Movement: "The Mission Is Nutrition"

Family Values?

Km is a liquid potassium/herbal preparation produced by Matol Botanical International Ltd. of Montreal, Canada. It is sold from person to person through distributors in many countries. I became curious about it in 1990 when a local distributor told me that one of her many satisfied customers was a patient with kidney disease and a chronically high blood potassium level. An observant Christian, this distributor called *Km* a "spiritual product." A few months later she invited me to a large public meeting and sponsored me as a distributor.

According to the August 1991 issue of Matol's *Journal*, the company's mission is:

> To impact World Health and the environment positively through products, services, education and programs that promote quality of life and healthy living; to impact the vision of humanity and the world we live in.

Matol's "governing values," listed below the mission statement, are: integrity, quality, leadership, independence, family, respect, financial security, loyalty, and personal growth. Independence, the statement suggests, can be achieved "by promoting and encouraging everyday health, wealth, self-esteem and freedom from unnecessary obligations, servitude and oppression." The September 1991 *Journal* carries a "message from the Matol partners" titled "Integrity is First," which defines integrity as "the

143

quality or state of being of sound moral principle with uprightness, honesty and sincerity." An article titled "Integrity—A Private Journey" begins on the next page. In a 1992 issue, Matol's co-founder, J.F. Robert Bolduc, describes Matol as a "mini-society" striving "to become the World's Health Corporation." "Our products," he writes, "have personalities of their own; they carry powers that exceed those of our individual efforts." A drawing in a later issue depicts a Matol distributor holding a bottle of *Km* in maternal fashion, with Henry Ford, Thomas Edison, and Alexander Graham Bell in the background.

"Destiny Intervened"

The history of *Km* is vividly described in company brochures and videotapes, which provide the following details.

Km was formulated in the 1920s by Karl Jurak, a student of agrobiology and biochemistry at the University of Vienna. In his youth, Karl was interested in flowers and plants and displayed an "unquenchable thirst for knowledge." One day while climbing a mountain he suddenly became weak and "dangerously short of breath." To improve his physical condition, he became "driven to establish a state of optimum health." He reasoned that "if he could find a way to focus his natural body energies, he would then find the key to relieving his problems. He decided to apply his knowledge of science and use the plants he loved . . . to prepare a health formula for himself."

Karl was "sure that nature had anticipated man's needs." After eight months of work, during which he analyzed his own blood samples daily, he arrived at a formula. But although he noted many benefits, the "key" to the formula was missing—"a factor that would perfectly merge all of the virtues of each plant." Finally, in 1922, the "key"—not specified in brochures—was revealed to him in a dream. He completed the formula and found that taking it led to "remarkable improvement." He based his doctoral thesis on this work and, at the age of nineteen, received a doctorate with honors in agrobiology. In 1925 he was awarded a second doctorate, in biochemistry.

In 1932, the story continues, the Canadian government commissioned Jurak to do research, and he emigrated to Canada. For thirty years he continued to prepare the formula himself. He did not sell it, but gave it to friends and relatives until, in 1962, he was no longer able to satisfy the demand and "destiny intervened." In that year Jurak entrusted the formula to his son, Anthony, who had earned his own doctorate in biochemistry. "But with the inheritance came the injunction not to change the formula."

Among the many persons using the privately prepared formula was a long-time friend of Jurak's son—J.F. Robert Bolduc. Bolduc, the manager of a market research firm in Montreal, became aware of the rapid growth of the natural products industry and the value of networking. In 1984, he and Anthony Jurak launched Matol Botanical International. Network marketing expert Sam Kalenuik joined them in 1986.

A 1989 brochure described Matol as a 150-million-dollar-a-year business. According to the July 1991 special edition of Matol's *Journal*, business was booming, with a volume increase of approximately 55 percent in the first quarter of the year.

An article by writer Kevin Krajick in the August 1989 issue of *Longevity* fills a few of the gaps in the above story. Initially, Matol Botanical International had a single product, *Matol*, which was marketed as a treatment for diseases ranging from rheumatism of the spine to prostate cancer. But Canada's Health Protection Branch (an agency similar to the FDA) eventually enjoined the company from making therapeutic claims for the product. Matol's attempt in 1985 to export its product to the United States was stymied by the FDA, which had it seized on grounds that extravagant claims rendered it an unapproved new drug. In April 1986, the FDA issued an Import Alert directing that shipments of *Matol* be detained. The company circumvented the FDA simply by adding cascara sagrada (a laxative) to its product and renaming it *Km*. (Recall Jurak's injunction against changing the formula.) In 1988, discovery of bacterial contamination prompted the recall of nearly 38,000 bottles of *Km*.

"Nauseating"

Km retails for $37.50 a quart and is packaged in a white plastic container bearing the words:

> a potassium mineral supplement preparation, in a non medicinal base, prepared by a special process from extracts of flowers, foliage, roots and barks of certain botanical plants. Km contains 585 mg of Potassium per serving of 2 tablespoons. Drink 1 tablespoon (15 ml) twice a day, morning and night, which can be mixed in milk or water.

The amount of potassium in each serving is not much more than the amount in eight ounces of orange juice or fruit-flavored lowfat yogurt, one broccoli stalk, or one medium-sized banana. However, Merlin Nelson, Pharm.D., a member of the National Council of Health Fraud, has observed that the actual amount of potassium in *Km* is unclear, since 585 mg of potassium can represent between 3.87 and 14.96 milliequivalents (mEq) of potassium. Most potassium prescription products furnish 8 mEq per dose.

The first three of the twenty-seven ingredients listed on the container—by far, the bulk of the product—are purified water, caramel color, and glycerin. Other ingredients include fourteen herbs, five minerals, and artificial flavors (unnamed except for vanillin, which was not in the original formula). Matol suggests that one ounce daily is appropriate for most people but that the dosage should be determined by how the user feels. In the January/February 1991 issue of *Nutrition Forum*, consumer advocate Stephen Barrett, M.D., said he had never tasted anything worse.

Km's label provides only the common names of its herbal ingredients; genus and species are not indicated, nor are the amounts. Furthermore, *Km* is not expiration-dated in the United States. The active constituents of herbs generally lose potency over time. Many are deactivated, for example, by heat and water. *Km* is mostly water, and my sponsor customarily stored it and other Matol products in the trunk of her car throughout the year. Thus, even ingredients that are potent when placed in the bottle might have no physical effect on the consumer. However, it is worth noting that four of them—chamomile, gentian root, senega root, and horehound—have been associated with nausea and/or vomiting.

A registered nurse told me my sponsor had sold her a bottle of *Km* with the claim that it would control her appetite. She said she had consumed it irregularly for about two to three weeks, but had been "very uncomfortable" because it was "nauseating." She further stated that it hadn't controlled her appetite and that she'd discarded the product. If *Km* can suppress appetite, the explanation may be that people tend not to eat when they are nauseous.

Matol's other products are more mundane. *FibreSonic*, the first of its "World Health Quest Products," is a powdered supplement featuring twenty-seven kinds of dietary fibers plus vitamins and minerals. The "Pathway Nutrition System," formerly called the "Pathway Program," is primarily a weight-management plan featuring meal-replacement shake powders and high-fiber meal-replacement bars. All Pathway products are marketed under the brand name *Matola*. The *Oat & Peanut Bars*, about two ounces each, sell for $21.00 per box of eight ($1.31 an ounce). These are similar to peanut butter-flavored *Slim-Fast* bars. Ounce for ounce, however, they were somewhat lower in protein, vitamins, and essential minerals than two types of *Slim-Fast* bars I purchased during 1991 and 1992. Yet the *Oat & Peanut Bars* cost over three times as much. My sponsor misrepresented them to me as fat-free.

Is there any good reason for choosing Matol's *Oat & Peanut Bars*? Yes, according to the original package: "Matol's Pathway Program fosters self-esteem, eliminates road blocks and strengthens personal intuition. This pathway to the realization of individual power, results in exciting lifestyle choices and personal development." The *Matola Bar* is a low-fat granola bar advertised as cholesterol-free, sweetened with honey and fruit juices, and containing "chelated minerals" and "certified organic ingredients." It also costs $21.00 per box of eight. Other Matol products include *Matola Cereal* and *Km Botanical Skin Care Lotion*. The latter is said to possess the "essential botanical properties" of *Km*.

A Pathway Advisory Board was introduced in 1992. Three of the four board members hold doctorates, including sports nutritionist Kristine Clark, a registered dietitian. In a *Journal* article, she indicates her family's credentials—e.g., two economics professors, a registered nurse, and a marathon runner—and then describes their reaction to trying *Matola* products. "I couldn't believe that all of my family was raving about the same thing at once," she writes. "But it was happening and I knew immediately that something unusually special surrounded these foods."

"Unpretentious Sharing": The Distributor's Kit

Multilevel marketing (MLM), also called network marketing, is a form of direct sales in which independent distributors sell products to their friends, acquaintances, and other contacts. Distributors can buy products wholesale, sell them at retail, and recruit others to do the same. Recruiters who enroll enough distributors become entitled to a percentage of their sales. Matol's sales pitch emphasizes financial opportunity as well as product integrity.

According to an article in the September/October 1991 issue of *Newlife*, a "New Age" magazine that focuses on "alternative" healthcare, "organizations based on hierarchy and domination" are being "superseded by a 'kinder, gentler' form that treats both employee and customer as friends." The article advocates MLM as a worthy and "fun" alternative to traditional employment and cites four MLM giants: Amway Corporation, Herbalife International, and Shaklee Corporation—all three of which market nutrient supplements—and Mary Kay cosmetics. The author, "intuitive counselor" Tom Goode, writes that there are over five million MLM distributors and that "MLM has produced more millionaires in the last twenty years than any other type of business by a large margin." (This "millionaire" story is part of MLM industry folklore but, as far as I know, it has never been documented.)

With no such financial illusions, I obtained my Matol distributor's kit by completing a simple application and paying my sponsor $90. The kit included a quart of *Km*, two ten-ounce packets of *FibreSonic*, a translucent measuring flask, a one-ounce measuring cup, a 1990 audiotape of an introductory talk by Sam Kalenuik, two slick videotapes, and a handsome loose-leaf binder. The binder contained product brochures and circulars, a sales receipt book, order forms, a *Prospecting & Sponsoring Handbook*, a *Distributor Manual*, a *Business Guide*, a catalog proffering Matol "designs" (e.g., clothing and accessories), an issue of Matol's *Journal* (published eight times a year), a question-and-answer booklet, record-keeping materials, a brochure requesting a donation to the nonprofit Dr. Karl Jurak Foundation (concerned with child abuse), and other paraphernalia. The box containing the kit bore the message: "I Am Staying Young. Ask Me How."

Matol's *Handbook* suggests using the following advertisement to attract new distributors:

> "Dissatisfied?" We are currently seeking 3 individuals with sales, management, or teaching backgrounds who have owned their own business. Must be capable of handling exceptionally large incomes. . . . Call for an appointment.

One day I observed my sponsor press an unemployed youth to become a distributor, assuring him that a distributorship was a "real job."

In the 1990 audiotape, Kalenuik states that Matol distributors number a quarter of a million. In the videotape entitled "An Idea Whose Time Has Come," the narrator says: "No important news flashes heralded the discovery [of *Km*], no documentation in prestigious journals—just an unpretentious sharing of human insight." One scene has a young boy denying his dog additional *Km*, unflinchingly downing an unmeasured amount and, as an afterthought, stuffing a second bottle of *Km* into his school bag. Another depicts a young girl about to "share" *Km* at school during "show-and-tell." Toward the end of the video, Karl Jurak, who turned eighty-eight in March 1992, tells us we "are the carriers of this important legacy."

The second videotape has three segments. In the first, "Building on

Destiny," Karl Jurak indicates that although he doesn't understand how *Km* works, it may "have something to do with purification and oxygenation of blood." The second segment consists mainly of testimonials from distributors about how enthusiastic they are and/or how much money they have made. Several state they have earned $30,000 per month, and Matol's top distributors, a married couple, are said to have made $82,579 in a single month. (The improbability of such earnings accruing to new distributors is not mentioned. My sponsor, who certainly marketed aggressively, told me that her income from Matol was about $700 per month.)

The third segment assures us that "Matol's phenomenal success is based on *Km* alone—no fancy packaging, no Madison Avenue hype. Just one single product that works." But the company also intends to "continue Dr. Jurak's dream in addressing the most pressing health problems facing mankind today. . . . obesity, environmental impurity, widespread dietary deficiency in both young and old. To meet these challenges, Matol introduces World Health Quest products. The first of these [*FibreSonic*] already promises to make a major contribution to international health."

Another video—"Why Herbs?"—was not part of the kit, but has been proffered by Matol as a sales aid. It asks us to "imagine a world sometime in the near future . . . where disease and other physical ailments have been virtually eradicated, where heart disease, high blood pressure, even cancer are no longer a threat." Such a situation will remain unlikely, says the narrator, until people take responsibility for their own health and stop relying on modern medicine—which "has failed miserably" and whose "cut-and-burn methods" are "deadly." Statistics are colorfully presented in support of the above view. What is the "simple and time-tested" answer to the "dilemma" of nutritionally inadequate food? This video says herbs—without which "good health is nearly impossible." And what is "the primary obstacle preventing herbs from reaching every home in America"? Fear, according to the video. "What is there to be afraid of?" asks the narrator. Better health? A longer life? Reduction of medical bills? The death of modern medicine? Simply beware, he says, of fraudulent products and disreputable manufacturers. No specifics are provided. In another video not included in the kit, titled "Pathway to Freedom," an unidentified "full-time health professional" and "doctor for thirty years" says that people should take *Km* "on a very regular basis."

Another sales aid, the *Pathway Research Manual*, gives elaborate instructions for combining foods to achieve what Matol considers the ideal balance of "alkaline-forming" and "acid-forming" foods. The average cost of Pathway products is said to be $19 to $50 per week (plus the cost of *Km*).

Bottled Hype

It is illegal for distributors to claim that *Km* is effective against any health problem. Matol's 1990 question-and-answer booklet states:

> We market our product as a food supplement and we do not make any therapeutic claims, but we do believe that most people can benefit from our product; this is why we are confident enough to offer a 30-day guarantee on the product.

Matol's *Journal* warns:

> An independent Matol Botanical International Ltd. Distributor is not permitted to diagnose or prescribe the products as a specific treatment for *any* disease or condition. To do so is likely in contravention of the law and is not condoned by Matol Botanical International Ltd.
>
> Matol Botanical International Ltd. does not make any claims whatsoever about its products and does not sanction or permit any of its Distributors to make any claims.

Although company literature makes no *direct* therapeutic claims for *Km*, one brochure provides pictures of its fourteen herbs and attributes beliefs about their usefulness to various peoples in the past. For example, it says that Indians of Virginia believed that passion flower could "quiet and soothe the body" and that native Indians on the Pacific coast of North America believed that tea made from saw palmetto berries "soothed and quieted the mind." Another brochure quotes Karl Jurak: "In 60 years, given time, I have never seen this product fail once in helping to do some good for the people using it."

It is clear that some distributors are making therapeutic claims. For example, some are circulating flyers or typed reports associating *Km*'s herbal ingredients with organs and health problems for which each herb can supposedly be of benefit. One such flyer, entitled "Herbal Information," refers neither to Matol nor to *Km*, but bears the handwritten name and phone number of the distributor and makes vague therapeutic claims for the herbs in *Km*. Alfalfa, for example, is described as "excellent for arthritis" and said to contain "many vitamins and minerals." A two-color circular touts *Km* as a "blood purifier" that has been "examined" for more than sixty years in the human body. Its message of "energy and vitality" and "a greater hope of longer life" comes through despite sloppy writing and eight misspellings. A 1992 issue of Matol's *Journal* acknowledges that such information is being circulated, citing unauthorized material titled "The Cancer Answer."

Have these and similar claims been scientifically tested? The question-and-answer booklet acknowledges:

> Other than those done by Dr. Karl Jurak way back in the beginning, no tests of any kind have been done. We do not believe that we will enter into any such programs since trying to prove what this product seems to have done for some people would be next to impossible. However, Matol's Km formula has been tested in the finest laboratory in the world for over 60 years—the human body.

The booklet also states that "if there were any contra-indications when using our products, the FDA would have instructed us to indicate that on our label. As you can see, the label does not carry any contra-indications.... If there are any side effects, they will appear briefly and will not be severe. These possible secondary effects could be manifested by diarrhea, constipation, lightheadedness, headache, itchy sensations, or nausea." The booklet concedes: "There have been all kinds of people seemingly allergic to something [in *Km*]." Nevertheless, discontinuation of use after such a reaction is not recommended.

Originally, my sponsor stated simply that the cost of *Km* is refundable. But later she added the stipulation that the buyer *consume* the product regularly for thirty days—even if he finds *Km* nauseating (as I did)! She also misinformed me regarding how I could subscribe to Matol's *Journal*, which she knew I was quite interested in receiving. Reciting the motto "a kit and a case," she advised me on a couple of occasions that I must purchase a case of *Km* in order to qualify for mailings of the *Journal*.

"New York Needs to Be Penetrated"

On February 13, 1991, I attended a two-hour Matol corporate meeting in the Grand Ballroom of the Holiday Inn adjacent to LaGuardia Airport in New York City. A banner above the podium advised in French and in English: "GIVE AND RECEIVE." The banner also showed a chart with a crooked line slanting upward at about 45 degrees. Below it stood two displays of Matol products.

Opening remarks were made by "executive advisor" Jacobus Jeffrey, who wore a green "2 FOR FREEDOM" button on his lapel. (The slogan refers to the strategy of "two in-home meetings a week for financial freedom.") My sponsor claimed that Mr. Jeffrey, whom she referred to as "Brother Jeffrey," was a member of the board of directors of Kingsbrook Jewish Medical Center in Brooklyn. She also said that "Matol meetings" were held there regularly in a conference room. However, in a phone conversation with me in September 1991, Martin Freiwirth, the chief executive officer of the center, denied that he knew anyone by the name of Jeffrey. Mr. Jeffrey is a trim-bearded, middle-aged, black, avowed New Yorker who speaks in measured tones. He welcomed an above-capacity, ethnically mixed crowd of well over 750 men, women, and children from New York and nearby states. The audience would grow to about 1,100.

Jeffrey stated that he was "so excited" about this long-awaited first New York corporate meeting. He asked all the nondistributors to raise their hands and then to stand up. Their rising was met with applause. "You are our guests," he told them. He promised all of us—twice—that we would not walk out as we had walked in, but would leave with a "different feeling."

Then he introduced chiropractor David Gordon from Bloomington, Indiana, as a "field advisor" and a "special, special person" who had made more than $100,000 in his first year with Matol. But before Gordon could commence his overview, Jeffrey said that he wanted to interject Matol's mission statement, and he articulated one of Matol's mottos: "Helping people to help people." At his request, the audience chanted the slogan. Jeffrey explained that the purpose of this meeting was to "build leaders in the tri-state and in the Matol family." "New York," he declared, "needs to be penetrated." Applause followed.

The Matol Distributor's Job: "To Tell Stories"

Jeffrey raised a copy of Matol's *Journal* above his head. Depicted on the cover were David Gordon and his wife, whom Jeffrey described as lovely. He made a fuss about how nice they were before inviting Gordon onto the podium. Gordon, who is short, assured us he was standing. He asked us how we were tonight ("Great!") and how our day had been (the same). He told us his suits were at the airport in Chicago, spoke of his prior depression, and reminisced about his boyhood summers in Buffalo, New York. Then he recounted the circumstances leading to his acceptance of *Km*.

"All you need to do," he advised, "is share the product with people and get them drinking it, and it'll do the work for you. Have you noticed that?" The applause suggested that the audience agreed. But he appeared disappointed with the response to his next question, regarding how many persons present were drinking *Km*.

"That's all?" he asked. "You've never had the joy of tasting it? . . .

You're in for a treat." He demonstrated the translucent measuring flask included in the distributor's kit, and advocated drinking *Km* from the flask in public to attract attention to the product.

Gordon said that "things started to happen" after he'd begun using *Km* in August 1989. Never a "morning person," for example, he had begun waking up two hours earlier than usual. After conveying his wife's negative opinion of the product's odor, he described *Km* as a potential "disaster" from a marketing standpoint. "So I tell people: it looks bad, it smells bad, it tastes bad, and it works." To which my sponsor responded, "Amen." (So did I—to myself. *Km* looks like an extract of mud and tastes vile!)

Gordon requested a show of hands from nondistributors who had come to "check out" Matol, and reacted with childish glee to the response. "This is a relationship business," he emphasized. He insisted that *Km* "works," and called attention to his family and educational backgrounds. He stated that his father had been a practicing physician, that his wife was a nurse, and that he himself had planned in high school to become a surgeon. He was thus, he said, a skeptic, and as such had approached the matter of *Km*.

When Gordon announced the upcoming establishment of an East Coast warehouse, the audience roared. He said that about three years earlier, *Km* had been temporarily unavailable and sold for $100 a bottle. "When you find out what's in that bottle," he explained, "you realize there isn't any price too high—if it's for someone you love." He further spoke of "integrity."

He described *Km* as a "universal product" from which anyone can derive benefit, and implied that it "would actually enhance oxygen efficiency to all sixty trillion cells of your body." The "remarkable responses" to *Km*, and their variety, he explained, are attributable to *Km*'s "working at the cellular level." Later, Gordon stressed that *Km* was both consumable and one of a kind. "We just happen to have a monopoly," he said.

What if *Km* doesn't "work"? "It takes time," he said. One-third of *Km* consumers allegedly recognize benefits (unspecified) within a few minutes to a few days of first using the product; another third within a week to a month; and another third within one to three months. According to a flyer: "The benefits of Km are immediate. But, the Km experience depends on a person's body awareness." The flyer identifies at least one alleged benefit: *Km* "facilitates . . . purification."

Gordon also talked about soil depletion: "We have stripped from our food supply 70 percent of the nutrients that should be available to us. We're trying to run . . . on 30 percent." Cells, he said, "get pooped" running on 30 percent. "Maybe you noticed how tired Americans are," he stated. He gave assorted statistics to support his sentiment that Americans are in bad shape.

Gordon summed up the Matol sales technique:

> The bottom line that we're sharing with people is results. That's it. The product works. . . . When you share stories of benefits with other people—not features of the product, [but] benefits . . . they will want to have it. When the perceived value of the product exceeds the cost, people will buy it. . . . Our job [is] to tell stories.

He stated that the "FDA has approved [*Km*] for use by everybody—men, women, children, [the] elderly, pregnant women, infants . . . heart patients. . . . It is a food supplement . . . a liquid salad." (In actuality, no products classed as "food supplements" are "approved" by the FDA.) *Km*, he said, "changes people physically, emotionally, psychologically, financially." He suggested that it can rehabilitate one's sense of humor.

Gordon claimed that the carbohydrate in the *Pathway* products "is in a time-release form, so you get a constant energy curve all day." He also claimed that the Pathway Program brings about loss of "just non-structural fat" and, furthermore, "actually sculpture[s] your body. . . . The weight comes off in the right places." But the Pathway Program, he counseled, won't work without *Km*, because "*Km* enhances the efficiency at the cellular level of utilization of all the nutrients." Moreover, he said, continued use of *Km* leads to better food choices: "You will desire better foods."

Gordon reported that sales hit $1.5 million one day around the time of a recent convention in Anaheim, California. He said February 1991 sales were projected to be nearly $20 million and that total 1990 sales had been nearly $200 million. Later he solicited testimonials from Pathway product users who had lost more than ten pounds. The four respondents reportedly had lost an average of one pound daily. When Gordon was through, Jacobus Jeffrey, joined by eighteen "achievers" on the podium, presided over a prolonged series of bilingual mutual and self-congratulations.

"A Sojourner Along the Way"

Then Jeffrey introduced Matol's "vice president of personal development," Dr. Clifford Baird (the "2 FOR FREEDOM" strategist), as a gentleman with "an educational background second to none." He explained that Baird had earned four traditional educational degrees and three others—in "life," mountaineering, and "streetology."

Baird, nearly 6 feet, 7 inches tall, told us how wonderful we and everything were, and identified his four degrees: a bachelor's in math, an M.A. in industrial psychology, an M.B.A. in banking and marketing, and a Ph.D. in psychology. Then he declared: "Wisdom is not the byproduct of education." Baird described himself at one point as "a sojourner along the way." His talk was filled with cliches. He struck me as a pop psychologist-preacher, but the audience responded to him with much laughter and applause. "You can walk into the basement of your fears," he concluded, "and put the lights on, and it's . . . not as bad as you thought it was."

Coffee, Tea, Me—or *Km*?

On April 10, 1991, I attended another "Opening of America" meeting, which drew some 2,000 people to the Radisson Hotel in Hauppauge, New York. A banner proclaimed 1991 "The Year of Freedom," and "New Age" music filled the hall prior to commencement. I had come by chartered bus with Mr. Jeffrey's group of thirty.

The opening speaker was John Paul Dadufalza, a 24-year-old of Philippine descent whose picture appears on the cover of Matol's July 1991 *Journal*. A former flight attendant, he had reportedly earned $20,265 in his fourth month as a distributor. My sponsor likened him to Michael Jackson. His somewhat exotic good looks and polished appearance in a tailored suit had made him the most conspicuous award recipient at the last meeting I'd attended. John Paul exuberantly recounted his gradual acceptance of *Km* and Matol, which he attributed to his mother's nagging. Unspecified "health challenges" finally prompted him to try *Km* six months after his mother had given him a bottle. However, he did not specify any benefit of *Km* other than financial. John Paul asked those who had lost weight on the Pathway program to stand, and called on the "big losers" to deliver testimonials.

I was disappointed to learn that the legendary Karl Jurak would not appear. Nor would Robert Bolduc. (My sponsor informed me he was busy pursuing a doctorate in network marketing.) But Anthony Jurak and Sam Kalenuik took turns on the podium.

"The Facts Don't Count"

Anthony Jurak told us it was his fifty-third birthday; he looked about ten years younger. He intimated a belief in destiny, and explained Matol's motto, "Give and receive": "We know for sure today that if you give, eventually you receive." Anthony did not quit with that maxim, adding: "If the dream is big enough, the facts don't count" and "Freedom is going on a holiday and not having a return ticket."

Kalenuik claimed he could tell us in twenty-five minutes or less how to get our lives in order, and announced two upcoming Matol products, including the *Matola Bar*, which he described as a chewy, high-fiber, low-fat bar made with all "organically grown" ingredients. He reiterated Anthony's saying about dreams and facts, expressed a strong desire "to have the biggest impact in two thousand years on world peace," and said that "you can dream as big as you want as long as you believe." He also expressed belief in the vitalistic, Jungian concept of "synchronicity": "Meaningful coincidences will occur in your life when you're headed in a right direction." Becoming increasingly metaphysical, he insisted: "Thoughts change matter. Thoughts *are* things." (This remark became the subject of a two-page photo layout in the September 1991 *Journal.*) Babies, he continued, have no limitations at all. Kalenuik thereupon inquired how many of us believed in God. About half the attendees raised a hand, but my sponsor assured me that the majority believed. Kalenuik told us we were all essentially equal, and that inequality results from wrong thinking.

Create Your Own Vitamins!

More mystifying was the local "Matol meeting" I attended at Kingsbrook Jewish Medical Center on the evening of October 1, 1991. Fourteen other people were present. My sponsor identified one of the attendees as a medical doctor and another as a detective. The latter gentleman wore a holster with a gun. Except for one young man, all appeared over fifty years of age. After a video presentation, a supervisor announced that Mr. Jeffrey would arrive late. Then he introduced the first speaker, who delivered a testimonial emphasizing economic rather than specific health benefits. "Eighty percent is the product," he stated, "twenty percent is you." He said that *Km* would soon be kosher and described the Pathway Program as "more than just *Slim-Fast*." His testimonial was followed by another speaker's tortuous expounding of the "marketing plan"—how to become a supervisor. My sponsor explained that the purpose of these meetings was to iron out the details of the distributors' relationship with the home office.

But such ironing out did not occur. Instead, the discussion descended into a babel of complaints, the most intelligible of which concerned the attendee's apparent inability to understand either the second speaker or the company's marketing plan.

Later, the supervisor claimed that "healthy bodies create their own vitamins." Another distributor restated this belief. The supervisor characterized distributors as "educators," but stated that it was not enough to be a "cerebral salesman." He said of *Km*: "The planet has never seen anything like this."

Jeffrey did not show up. He was, however, present at a Matol meeting held at Kingsbrook on February 4, 1992. Paula Manceri, a reporter for the television newsmagazine "Inside Edition," attended this meeting with a hidden camera. She informed me that discussion of economic concerns again predominated, and that Jeffrey was not a member of Kingsbrook's board of directors.

The Bottom Line

Matol and *Km* epitomize the "New Age" quest for a nutritional quick fix. Glittering generalities and "unauthorized" therapeutic claims aside, *Km* has never been proven safe or effective for any health purpose whatsoever. The identity and amounts of its herbal ingredients are not public information. Those who feel or look better after using *Km* are encouraged to attribute any improvement to the product's supposed potency. Those who feel worse are asked to persevere or change the dosage. These simple tactics—plus the lure of easy money—have enabled Matol to pull the wool over the eyes of a multitude of people from all walks of life.

11

The Shady Business of Nature's Sunshine

Out of the Kitchen

Nature's Sunshine Products, Inc. (NSP) is a network marketing organization headquartered in Spanish Fork, Utah. According to its literature, the company has grown from a "kitchen table enterprise" in 1972 into an international business with distributors in all fifty states, Canada, England, Australia, and New Zealand. The business began with herbs, but has expanded into nutritional supplements, homeopathic remedies, skin and hair-care products, water treatment systems, cooking utensils, and a weight-loss plan. Over the years, more than a quarter of a million people have signed on as "independent" NSP distributors. The company now markets over 175 herbal preparations among its more than four hundred products. For the first six months of 1992, its reported sales were $46.7 million, with net income of $2.4 million.

The Distributor Kit

Becoming a distributor requires no prior training in either health or nutrition—only submission of a one-page application and payment of a $35 fee.

NSP's distributor kit consists of a wire-bound book called *A Systems Guide to Natural Health* and a loose-leaf binder labeled "The People-To-People Health Business." The latter contains a congratulatory form letter, a product catalog, a policies and procedures manual, four different price lists, distributor applications, order forms, a receipt book, and flyers concerning products, payment plans, discounts for new distributors, and group insurance.

The form letter states: "Less expensive products are available from competitors and may appear similar; however, these products are often formulated down to a price, rather than up to a standard." It refers to benefits such as "holistic health insurance" for managers. "Herb combinations," according to the product catalog, "take advantage of the synergistic properties inherent in herbs to achieve superior nutritional impact. Thus, a combination of herbs can often address a broad spectrum of nutritional needs unsatisfied by a single herb alone." In contrast, the "sidebar" begins in boldface: "saponins, oils, alkaloids and esters, that's what herbs are made of." The catalog states that NSP's Chinese herbal combination products are based on the "five element model" and on the principles of yin and yang.

The policies and procedures manual features a 15-point code of ethics, which includes: "I will not make any false or therapeutic claims concerning any NSP product" and "I will service a minimum of ten retail customers each month." The manual also states: "If a customer asks for permission to return a product that he/she is dissatisfied with, verify that it has been used for a reasonable length of time." Distributors are advised to separate "educational" and sales or recruiting activities. They are further advised against conducting herb lectures where products or sales aids are stored. The apparent purpose of this advice is to encourage distributors to make claims in their lectures that could create legal difficulty for the company if placed on product labels.

The *Systems Guide,* published in 1988, contains about eighty pages. About half of the book describes various body systems and the products NSP relates to them. For each system, there are "key," "primary," and "complementary" products. Key products combine ingredients to "provide comprehensive nutritional support" for the body system. Primary products are combinations "designed to provide more specialized support for the particular system." Complementary products are single-ingredient items "for individuals who want to round out the systems approach to holistic health." These products include acidophilus, aloe vera, cascara sagrada (a laxative), and magnesium.

The circulatory system's key product is *Mega-Chel*, which contains twelve vitamins, nine chelated minerals, choline, inositol, PABA, bioflavonoids, fish oils, adrenal substance, thymus substance, and spleen substance. The "primary" circulatory products include *CoQ-10 Plus*;

Bugleweed Liquid Herb; *Capsicum, Garlic & Parsley*; and herbal mixtures (*BP-X, GC-X, GGC, ATC, HS-II*, and *I-X*) that contain from three to fourteen ingredients. The complementary products include butcher's broom root, capsicum, garlic, hawthorn berries, liquid chlorophyll, magnesium, omega-3 fatty acids, and yellow dock root. Each of these products is said to provide "nutritional support" for the circulatory system. Products for other body systems are listed in the following table:

Body System	Key Products	Claims for Key Product
Circulatory	Mega-Chel	Improves vascular and heart muscle tone; improves circulation throughout the body; lowers LDL
Digestive	Food enzyme digestive aid Protein digestive aid (HCl)	Enhances utilization of food; supports weakened pancreas For people who need help digesting protein or are on a high-protein diet
Intestinal	Bowel Build	Nutritionally enhances digestion and provides dietary fiber; promotes cleansing of toxic intestinal buildup
Nervous	Nutri-Calm	Provides the nutrition the body needs to cope with a busy modern world
Glandular	Master Gland Formula	Strengthens the thyroid, adrenals, and pancreas
Immune	Immune Maintenance Formula	Counters the effects of poor foods, pollution, and other harmful things
Respiratory	ALJ Formula	Removes toxins trapped in mucous linings of the respiratory system
Structural	SKL Formula Target Endurance Formula	Maintains strong and healthy bones Nutritionally feeds the body's muscles
Urinary	URY	Nutritionally supports the urinary system; helps cleanse the blood and increase resistance to infection
Skin and Hair	External: Herbal Trim Internal: HSN-W	Works from the outside in to break up and rid the body of toxins and impurities Nutritionally supports the structure and function of the skin from within

Body Hype

Since 1989, NSP has been marketing *GlanDiet,* a meal-replacement program based mainly on the book, *Dr. Abravanel's Body Type and Lifetime Nutrition Plan* (1983), by Elliot B. Abravanel, M.D., and his wife Elizabeth King. The book maintains that there is a "dominant gland" at the root of every weight problem and that weight can be controlled by soothing the errant gland and moderating its cravings. The book advises that the corrective plan be tailored to the individual's "body type," which is determined by examining the person's shape, body fat distribution, food cravings, sleep patterns, and various other characteristics. Women can be classified as "thyroid," "pituitary," "adrenal," or "gonadal" type, while men can be classified as "thyroid," "pituitary," or "adrenal." The personality traits described for each type resemble those of a typical horoscope.

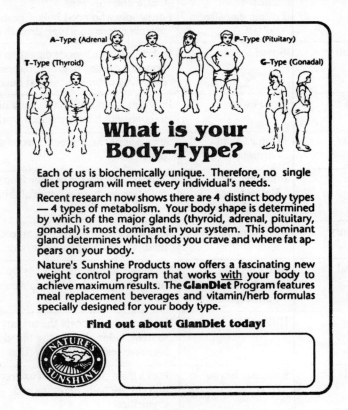

Advertising slick for GlanDiet (1990)

GlanDiet ads distinguish body types according to body shape and fat distribution: thyroid types gain weight in their midsection (acquiring a "spare tire"); gonadal types, in the hips, thighs, and buttocks; adrenal types, throughout the trunk or midsection; and pituitary types, throughout the body in the form of "baby fat."

"The object of the GlanDiet Program," according to a pamphlet, "is to bring balance to out-of-balance systems." Two kinds of meal-replacement powders are available. The one formulated for thyroid and pituitary types is said to contain more protein than carbohydrate "because carbohydrates tend to stimulate the pituitary and thyroid glands, while protein tends to stimulate the adrenals and gonads." The other kind, formulated for adrenal and gonadal types, is said to have a higher ratio of carbohydrate to protein.

To help distributors design the correct program, NSP provides "a convenient body type questionnaire . . . based solely upon shape and build." *GlanDiet* guidelines list "foods to eat or avoid" and "herbs to use when the urge to snack strikes" for each body type. All dieters are advised to begin with a two- to three-day "cleanse," engage in aerobic exercise, and aim for an overall calorie count of 1,200/day for women or 1,400/day for men. Of course, most people who exercise and restrict calories to such levels will lose weight whether or not they use NSP products.

"Homeopathic" Products

Homeopathy is based on the idea that greatly diluted substances can have powerful therapeutic effects on the body. Homeopathy's originator, Samuel Hahnemann, also believed that all chronic ailments have three sources: syphilis, venereal warts, and *psora* (Greek for "itch"). These ideas are utter nonsense, but the FDA permits homeopathic products to be marketed without proof that they work as claimed. NSP markets more than fifty homeopathic products, most of which are named after a disease or symptom. The product *Parasites,* for example, is said to be for "minor intestinal symptoms associated with parasites such as bloating, abdominal pain, flatulence and diarrhea." The product *Gout* is for "minor pain, heat, redness, and swelling associated with gouty inflammation of the joints." *Incontinence* is for "occasional minor bladder incontinence (involuntary urination) in adults." *Depressaquel* is designed "to assist in the reduction of minor feelings of melancholy, apathy and listlessness by lifting the mood and mental outlook." And so on. Each product contains minute amounts of about ten ingredients.

An NSP manual depicts the label of each homeopathic product on a separate page, followed by long lists of symptoms said to be associated with each ingredient. For example, *Gout* contains a 1:100,000 dilution of poison ivy, which is "associated" with "rheumatic and gouty conditions which worsen in cold, wet weather, improve with movement." The manual also lists "nutritional support companion products" for many of the homeopathic products. This setup enables NSP to suggest therapeutic uses for herbal products and supplements without making explicit claims for them.

The July 1992 issue of NSP's *Horizons Bulletin* states: "Because only minute dilutions of the original substance remain in a homeopathic remedy, side effects are almost unknown. No one knows just how such dilutions work, but thousands of people attest to their effectiveness. . . . [including] singer Tina Turner and actress Lindsay Wagner." It further states:

> Homeopathy enjoys formal recognition as a branch of medicine under federal law. Homeopathic remedies, considered over-the-counter medications by the FDA, are available without prescription, and are specifically designed to remedy common self-diagnosable conditions.

This statement is only partly true. The FDA has not "recognized" homeopathy "as a branch of medicine." A provision of the 1938 federal Food, Drug, and Cosmetic Act recognized substances listed in the *U.S. Homeopathic Pharmacopeia* as drugs. The recognition was an act of Congress spearheaded by a senator who was a homeopathic physician. It was not based on scientific evidence of effectiveness, but was a political decision.

Although the FDA could require that homeopathic remedies be proven effective in order to remain on the market, it has not chosen to do so. FDA enforcement officials do not believe that homeopathic remedies are effective therapeutic agents. They have merely made a political decision to ignore them unless they are marketed for the treatment of cancer or other serious diseases.

FDA regulatory guidelines state that "nonprescription homeopathics may be sold only for self-limiting conditions recognizable by consumers" and that their labeling "must adequately instruct consumers in the product's safe use." Parasites, depression, gout, incontinence, and several other conditions for which NSP markets products do not appear to meet these criteria.

Dubious Diagnostics

Iridology and an unscientific form of muscle-testing are utilized as a basis for recommending NSP products. Iridology is a pseudoscience, according to which one's health status can be appraised by examining the iris (the colored portion of the eye surrounding the pupil). Iridologists claim to diagnose "imbalances" that can be corrected with vitamins, minerals, herbs, and similar products. In *Iridology Simplified* (1980), which is on NSP's suggested reading list, chiropractor Bernard Jensen states: "By knowing in advance one's weak tissues and organs, as can be revealed by iridology, it is possible to supply needed nutrients and thereby prevent unnecessary illness and disease from occurring."

Muscle-testing is the "centerpiece" of an elaborate vitalistic system of diagnosis and treatment called "applied kinesiology" (AK). This should not be confused with kinesiology, which is the scientific study of muscles and bodily movement. AK originated as a diagnostic method in the mid-1960s with Michigan chiropractor George Goodheart, who theorized that muscle groups share "energy pathways" with internal organs; thus every organ dysfunction is discoverable in a related muscle. Testing muscles for relative strength and tone supposedly taps the body's "innate intelligence" and enables practitioners (most of whom are chiropractors) to detect specific dysfunctions. In *Applied Kinesiology: Muscle Response in Diagnosis, Therapy, and Preventive Medicine* (1987), Tom and Carole Valentine write: "If you'd like to have some fun, create some bumper stickers that read: 'Wobbly hips mean lousy nutrition,' or 'better femoral angulation for better night vision.'"

One stated goal of AK muscle-testing is to detect nutritional deficiencies and intolerance to specific foods. One type of testing is done after food substances have been placed in the mouth to produce salivation. If the muscles being tested are determined to be "strong," the substance is deemed beneficial for the organs associated with those muscles. If they are determined to be "weak," the substance is judged harmful.

AK is complicated, however, by the variety of muscle-testing methods. In *Health and Healing* (1983), "alternative" medicine proponent Andrew Weil, M.D., cites it as "a technique whose ready acceptance disturbs me." He writes:

> The [AK] practitioner might ask the patient to extend an arm and resist downward pressure. The test is repeated as the patient puts the other hand on and off different areas of the body or as

substances such as salt, sugar, and various drugs are placed on the body. Decrease in resistance of the arm muscles is supposed to signal internal problems at those areas or prove the harmfulness for that patient of the substances tested.

Weil concludes that AK "looks to me very much like a suggestive phenomenon." In fact, several controlled studies have found no difference in responses to test substances and placebos. Although AK is essentially a diagnostic method, it has come to embrace a variety of dubious modalities, including acupuncture, acupressure, and supplementation.

During my investigation of Nature's Sunshine, I did not ascertain the precise manner in which its distributors use iridology and muscle-testing to market their wares. Regardless of the details, under state laws, a commercial interaction in which a person attempts to discover a health problem and recommends a product to solve it constitutes the practice of medicine. NSP is well aware of this fact. Its literature and training sessions warn distributors not to "diagnose" or "prescribe." The distributor application form requires an acknowledgment that NSP's products "are not intended for and are not to be sold as a cure, ameliorant or palliative for any disease or ailment, and that such products are sold solely and only for nutritional purposes." An article in the February 1989 issue of *Sunshine Horizons* advises distributors:

Teach, don't prescribe and diagnose. . . .
Instead of diagnosing, ask questions. Be particularly careful when using iridology and muscle testing. For instance, don't say "You have a sinus problem." Rather, ask them, "Do you have sinus problems?" Let them diagnose themselves. You can also teach by talking to them in the third person. For example, you might say, "People with lymphatic rosaries typically have trouble with their sinuses." Or you can cite authorities: "Dr. Bernard Jensen says that this particular eye sign is associated with sinus congestion."
Always make clear that the information you are providing is only educational in nature and that the decision as to what they will do must be left up to them. . . .
Practice saying things correctly with family and friends so that the correct things to say and do are so ingrained in you that you never have to worry about getting "trapped" into practicing medicine without a license, even when dealing with strangers.

Despite the doubletalk, this approach appears illegal. Courts have long ruled that one cannot escape responsibility for practicing medicine without a license or marketing an unapproved drug by calling the practice or drug something else. In addition, the use of false statements to sell products constitutes theft by deception.

My sponsor's manager, a former plumber, said that in tough cases he relied on *The How-To Herb Book* (1984), recommended by NSP. The book specifies "basic herbs for pregnancy" and "remedies for common problems of pregnancy," including anemia, uterine hemorrhages, "false labor," miscarriage, stretch marks, and toxemia. "Herbs work well for babies," the book states, because "babies' immune systems haven't been hindered by lots of drugs" (they thus "respond quickly") and because "herbs have no side effects." Specific herbs and vitamins are recommended for over a dozen children's illnesses, including jaundice. One chapter deals exclusively with the herbal and nutritional treatment of about a hundred ailments, including alcoholism, baldness, cataracts, diabetes, gangrene, hepatitis, hyperactivity in children, impotence, mononucleosis, nephritis, intestinal obstruction, Parkinsonism, and senility.

Distributor Training

NSP sponsors many meetings and courses at which distributors can be trained.

• Distributor School is a two-day program given at various locations throughout the United States and open to all distributors and managers. In 1988, NSP launched the program and announced:

> Distributor School will be built around the new catalog, "A Systems Guide to Natural Health." Students will learn [NSP's] philosophy of natural health, plus they will be taken on a tour of the body, system by system. For each system they learn the basics of what that body does and what happens when it starts to break down. Attendees will come away actually knowing the key products to use for each of these systems. Thus they will have a working knowledge of which nutritional supplements to choose to feed the various systems of the body.
>
> In addition, there will be a carefully constructed business and motivation session that will teach distributors how they can support their own good health habits by sharing their new-found knowledge with others.

NSP's Distributor School kit provides specific guidelines for staying within the law and proposes "legal" ways to promote NSP supplements, such as discussing the "historical uses" of herbs and how herbs, "as foods," contribute to health. According to the kit, NSP will pay up to $2,000 per calendar year to help defray the expenses of any lawsuit filed against active distributors or managers on grounds of prescribing or diagnosing.

• Manager School was a five-day program given several times a year at the company's home office. Its purpose was to train people to "really be Natural Health Counselors." The program included "in-depth training in iridology, muscle-testing and nutritional supplements," with "business and legal information . . . woven into the fabric of how to actually practice natural health consulting properly." The program also included role-playing of counseling sessions. The course materials included iridology and muscle-testing charts. Managers were encouraged to hold regular meetings to explain the body systems and key products to new distributors. In late 1991, Manager School was converted into a two-day affair called Natural Health and Business School.

• A Professionalism Symposium is offered following the company's national convention each year. This meeting features speakers on health and business topics and workshops on muscle-testing, advanced iridology, Chinese herbology, and new NSP products.

• Other educational opportunities are offered through area herb conferences, lectures at the national convention, conferences for leading distributors, and regional conferences for distributors who wish to focus on selling NSP's water treatment systems.

Distributor School

In the spring of 1992, I contacted NSP's Manager Service Department via its toll-free number and expressed an interest in becoming a distributor. The department referred me to a potential sponsor residing in my neighborhood, whom I phoned. This distributor was Spanish-speaking and evinced a limited comprehension of English. At one point, his son explained that the distributor had to see a "patient"—whereupon I inquired if the distributor was a doctor. The son replied that he was an iridologist.

On April 4, 1992, I attended NSP's Distributor School, held in an amphitheater at the Marriott Hotel and Conference Center in Uniondale, Long Island, New York. The tuition was $35. Fifty-eight people were registered that morning. The *Distributor School Preparatory Workbook* states the goal of the school: "To provide an active understanding of Natural Health which can be used to improve health and can be shared with family and friends." According to the February/March 1991 issue of *Sunshine Horizons*, this school—"the foundation of NSP education"—has trained more than 2,000 distributors.

The program began with a video titled "Why Herbs?" which promoted herbal supplementation in general. Shortly after this presentation, Molly Wright, our "trainer," said she wanted "to talk about where health begins." She asked us where we thought it begins, and told us to feel free to answer her questions. A distributor responded: "On the cellular level."

"The millions and millions and billions of cells" of which the body is composed, said Molly, have five basic needs: (1) oxygen, (2) water, (3) nutrients, (4) proper elimination, and (5) even temperature.

"About how long did people used to live?" she asked. "Can you remember?" She cited the biblical patriarch Methuselah, reputed to have lived 969 years. "So that was when?" she asked. "The very beginning of the world. What kind of environment did they have? [Methuselah] was the oldest, but there were other people who lived in the hundreds of years and were still having children after they were hundreds of years old. That's very hard for us to imagine. So why did they live so long? Why can you suppose that they lived so long?"

The distributors' responses included: (1) superior nutrition, or as Molly put it, "a more pure form of nutrition"; and (2) a lower level of stress. One distributor explained that people had lost such longevity after the "great flood of Noah," which, he said, had weakened the atmosphere. Progressive defects in the Noachic bloodline, he argued, had thus resulted from an increase in exposure to solar radiation. Molly termed this "an interesting point."

She stated that we can "control a certain amount" of the body's five basic needs. "What we can control," she said, "it's our business to try to control." She described herbs and vitamins as "a great nutritional source," particularly "when we eat foods that don't have all the nutritional value." Then she referred to Alexis Carrel (1873-1944), a French-American surgeon who had received the 1912 Nobel Prize for Medicine. Carrel developed methods for keeping tissues and organs alive in vitro for long periods. Citing this work, Molly suggested that strict direction of the cellular environment is necessary for optimal health. The workbook also cites Carrel and states: "Under proper conditions, cells can live forever."

In 1911, the *Journal of the American Medical Association* published an article by Carrel, in which he briefly described his experiments. He wrote:

It may easily be supposed that senility and death of tissues are not a necessary phenomenon and that they result merely from accidental causes, such as accumulation of catabolic substances and exhaustion of the medium. The suppression, then, of these causes should bring about the rejuvenation of the arrested culture and thus increase considerably the duration of its life. . . .

The rejuvenation consists in removing from the culture substances that inhibit growth and in giving to the tissue a new medium of development.

However, Carrel specified in the article that aging and death were unnecessary only "under the conditions and within the limits of the experiments." In his internationally famous experiment, a fibroblast from an embryonic chicken heart apparently lasted thirty-four years in vitro before the culture was discontinued. But researchers have cast doubt upon this experiment, speculating that the culture was contaminated with fresh cells. In any case, present-day investigators have been unable to keep most cells alive in vitro beyond a certain number of generations.

"If you've ever been to a nutrition class in the medical university," Molly said, "the nutrition specialist will say that you really don't need vitamins and herbs because if you eat the right foods . . . you'll get the right nutrients you need. But we can't trust all the foods we're eating. . . . We can't always rely on the quality. . . . The quality of the nutrients . . . is certainly important."

This "lack of nutrients," according to Molly, causes a "weakening condition" of the body. "Another way that the body gets sick," she said, is "toxic buildup." This, she claimed, is caused by "a stressful environment and improper elimination." Then she mentioned Chinese yin-yang philosophy.

"When the body is trying to accumulate its nutrients," Molly elucidated, "if it's clogged with toxins, then . . . even if you're giving it all the right things, it's not going to be able to use them as it should because of this toxic condition." She expounded:

Anytime you're talking with somebody new about . . . natural health and trying to use health prevention . . . you're going to need to look at the cleansing place first. And what would happen if we never cleaned our home? Dust, cobwebs, everything [would] pile up. I mean, if we didn't have any kind of cleansing procedure going on, we can see visually what would happen. . . . That same type of thing happens in your body. . . . After everything it's been exposed to . . . if . . . after a period of time it weakens and it's not able to eliminate properly like it should, those toxins are going to build, and so we need to assist it in cleaning.

"Nature's Spring"

Next, Molly discussed tap water safety. "Why," she asked, "don't we think they clean it to the purest drinking form?" A distributor answered: "It costs money." Molly agreed:

> We probably already pay enough in taxes, and it would just cost a lot more to make sure that all of our water that is supplied to us in our homes is suitable for drinking. . . . Most of the water that is supplied to your home is not used for drinking. . . . And so, the solution then would be to clean just the water that you're going to drink. And since the city can't do that for us at this time, we need to be aware of how we can best do that.

Molly told us that the solution to tap-water problems is *Nature's Spring II*, an NSP water treatment system retailing for $520. In a video presentation that followed, the narrator described it as "an easy-to-use countertop unit designed to help ensure that the water you drink is the way nature intended it to be." A distributor in my row informed Molly that she'd had her tap water tested and that "the results were really shocking." She said the sample had contained fecal matter and had been "very toxic, very high in metals, very high in lead." I later observed this distributor washing down some pills with what she said was "Nature's Spring" water. She had brought a gallon container of it with her.

"The difference in the taste—that's kind of interesting," said Molly. "It does to me taste a lot better because I'm used to it now. But when we first bought our *Nature's Spring* unit, I put the regular tap water and then the *Nature's Spring* clean water in two different cups, and I had my husband taste it to see which one he liked better; and he picked the one that was regular tap water."

Another distributor expressed concern over the quantity of water potentially wasted—four to nine gallons per gallon of treated water, according to Molly. Molly replied that "it's certainly up to the individual if you want to retain that water and use it for other things that you normally use water for," and supported use of the unit:

> You can think of it . . . in the content [sic] of: you're using this [potentially wasted] water to clean the water that you need for your

body. You'll wash your vegetables when you come home from the produce store. You'll wash your fruit that you eat. . . . So you're always washing things for your body. What about washing the water for the inside of your body? That's the important place to start.

Later, she explained:

Think of material that can get into your water supply from the aquifers where the water comes from or from the reservoirs, or wherever your water is coming from. Whatever's put into that water, whatever's in the environment can be absorbed in that water, from the rainfall, whatever's in the sky . . . . Insecticides, pesticides . . . even the things that are used to treat the water are harmful for you. . . . The Environmental Protection Agency—the EPA—recognizes 1,110, I think, pollutants that are in the average drinking water supply. . . . And then the American Cancer Society comes in and says: out of that list, they find that 190 of those [pollutants] are linked to cancer. And then, out of [the total] . . . only thirty . . . are treated by the city's water treatment system.

NSP's brochure for its water-treatment devices states that distributors are independent of the company and "not authorized to make any representations on behalf of Nature's Sunshine." The brochure also states:

Nothing in this material or in any statement concerning Nature's Sunshine, or in any statement attributed to Nature's Sunshine, is intended to make any of the following representations, claims, or statements: (1) That your water supply contains, or may contain, any contaminant or contamination (or any health-related physical, chemical, biological, or radiological substance or matter); (2) That scientific certainty exists regarding the relationship between acute or chronic illness and water supply.

In response to a question, Molly stated that the unit's "membrane" has "about a year life span." It retails for $146. Although the unit includes a "pre-filter," Molly said that some users add another to the unit, "because of certain things that they're aware of in their water." The pre-filter retails for $50. One distributor reported that his unit had lasted only for about two months, and that he had returned it for a replacement. "The pre-filter," he explained, "got clogged very fast." He said he had installed an additional pre-filter in the replacement unit, but that the problem had recurred nonetheless.

(Water safety is a complex issue. Unsafe water usually tastes all right. The most problematic drinking-water pollutants, according to the January

1990 *Consumer Reports,* are lead, radon, and nitrate. Testing water for lead is inexpensive, and there are two simple measures to reduce levels: letting the water run for about a minute, and using only cold water. Testing water for radon is also inexpensive. The likeliest sources of water-borne radon are private wells and small-community water systems; rivers, lakes, and reservoirs are not likely sources. And private wells in farming communities are the likeliest source of water-borne nitrate.)

Cool Down and "Clean Out the Dirty"

After a break, Molly discussed NSP's herbal "supplements" and two books written and published by chemist Mark Pedersen, whom she identified as NSP's director of research and development. The books, which sold for about $12 each, were *Nutritional Herbology* (1991) and *Nutritional Herbology, Volume II: Herbal Combinations* (1990).

The back cover of the first volume states that *Nutritional Herbology* "provides the nutritional profile or 'label' for 106 commonly used herbs and natural foods. It is ironic that avid 'label readers' are only provided nutritional profiles of processed foods, while the most desirable foods, natural herbs, foods and food supplements are never sold with nutritional information, until now." But, according to the cover, the book "combines a detailed history and use of each herb with the nutritional profile to explain and interpret many historical uses of herbs as foods and medicines." Actually, Pedersen goes further in his book, listing: (1) herb constituents of little or no nutritional import, (2) the "definite actions" and "probable actions" of each herb, and (3) instructions on preparation and dosage. *Nutritional Herbology* categorizes herbs according to what Pedersen considers their active constituents:

1. Aromatic—volatile oils
2. Astringent—tannins
3. Bitter—phenolic compounds, saponins, or alkaloids
4. Mucilaginous—polysaccharides
5. Nutritive (foodstuffs)

In the introduction to the second volume, Pedersen describes his classification system as empirical, "integrating the classical four-element model of the universe with active chemical constituents." (He doesn't explain what happened to the fifth element mentioned in other NSP materials.) Volume two categorizes herbal combinations according to the physiological system for which they are purported to be therapeutic: circulatory, digestive, glandular, etc. The combinations are further classified according to whether they are recommended for "excess conditions" or for "deficient conditions." Volume two includes a "medical index" of diseases and symptoms.

Molly cited Pedersen as responsible for many of NSP's herbal combination products. She expounded:

> He has written books to give . . . information on Nature's Sunshine Products. And Nature's Sunshine cannot sell these books, even though they're perfect for our use, because we're a manufacturing company and [we] realize the conflict between a manufacturing company and a publishing company. The FDA recognizes that as conflict of interest, [and so] we can't publish the information that you really want to know about the products. We can only do one because of the legal implications there. We can't look like we're prescribing actual products that we're manufacturing. So that's why we have such a healthy education program, and everyone is into self-learning . . . because we have to learn about this somewhere and we have to start somewhere. So, these books are a really good source.

Molly thereupon announced that the books could be bought from her and briefly described the first volume. "When you put these herbs together in certain combinations," she claimed, "they actually go in and target and help with whatever's going on." Her assertions were based on Pedersen's empirical classification system. The Distributor School kit lists four categories of herbs: (1) aromatic herbs, said to "stimulate action, speed things up"; (2) mucilaginous herbs, said to "soothe, lubricate, absorb water/toxins, slow things down"; (3) bitter herbs, said to "loosen, soften, relax, dissolve, liquefy"; and (4) astringent herbs, said to "contract, tighten, tense, tonify, solidify tissue."

Molly cited several herbs, including aloe vera and slippery elm, as mucilaginous. "A mucilage herb has a cooling down effect," she told us. "It has a soothing effect." She claimed that aloe vera "has cooling properties in it" and would have a cooling effect on "the inflammation in the body or whatever needs to be cooled down in the body." "If you have anything hot before [ingesting] slippery elm," she stated, "then you will feel that cooling down going on." She said that saponins, present in bitter herbs, may be thought of as soap, since they "clean out the dirty." Her description of astringent herbs dovetailed with Pedersen's empirical system:

Astringent herbs have an active ingredient which is acid. . . . A lemon is acidic, and when you bite into a lemon, what do you do? You pucker. That acid squeezes and makes you pucker, and it makes you salivate more, because if you pucker, it just dries you up. So you salivate more to compensate for that. That puckering is a tightening that's going on, and . . . the acid ingredients in the herbs have a tightening effect. So in your function of this classification of herb, we have tightening, or toning, or building. All of these types of things come from the astringent properties.

She cited uva ursi as an astringent herb: "It's used as a natural diuretic, okay? Think of what a diuretic is doing."

Both a "key product" and a "systems product," *Bowel Build* is a combination of vitamins, minerals, herbs, and digestive enzymes. NSP's catalog describes it as "food for the gastrointestinal tract itself." Molly said it was a good example of a synergistic product, having both "laxative-type herbs in it to help cleanse" and "building-type herbs in it to help strengthen the . . . system." She asked if they would "cancel each other out," and then explained that "the herbs work not like a chemical or a drug that's going to actually change something. They're just going to either . . . support or cleanse the system somehow so that it gives you the right benefit." The herbs will do "what's needed," she claimed, but "won't have any bad effect on the rest [of the system]."

Prescribing v. Recommending

The "systems approach" was Molly's next topic. She began with the digestive system. "This," she said, "is where you should start when you're thinking about health . . . . Cleansing is very important because . . . if you want to give yourself nutrients that your body needs and there are toxins blocking the way for those nutrients to be used, then you need to clean those toxins out of the way first so that you can use those nutrients."

A distributor asked whether NSP carried a comfrey-pepsin combination. Molly replied that the company had offered this combination, but that it had been replaced with a marshmallow-pepsin combination because "they found that that one worked better." However, the price lists I obtained at the school refer to a comfrey-pepsin product. Comfrey can contain compounds that are toxic to the liver and have a cumulative effect. Both root and leaf of the plant have been found to cause cancer in rats fed relatively small amounts. What herbalist Steven Foster concludes in the February/March 1992 issue of *The Herb Companion* is more to the point:

"I will refrain from ingesting it, and I suggest you do the same."

"If you are working with your medical doctor on something that you have a specific problem with," Molly told a questioner, "I don't want you to—I'm not advocating that you stop doing that. But you can use your judgment and your education. . . . The drugs are going to probably cause the herbs to not work like they should." Later, she stated: "Some drugs will wipe out the effects of your herbs." Although Molly advised distributors who were not licensed health professionals against prescribing or diagnosing, she did suggest an alternative:

> If somebody comes to you . . . or if you know somebody who has friends with, like, a diabetic problem, [who have not seen] their physician, who would give them insulin, then—then, you use your knowledge about the product that would support somebody with a diabetic condition. And you recommend to them that that's what you would do if you had that type of condition in the body.

Molly rationalized:

> You're giving a referral, basically, just like you would recommend a movie that you saw or a play that you saw and that you enjoyed. You're telling them that you had that experience, and you're telling them about the experience that you had with this product, and that's why it would work. And if you don't know of [any] experience, you can do some research into the historical uses, and they need to rely on the historical uses.

The "Herbal Hour"—a home meeting designed to generate sales—is described in printed material I obtained at the school. It includes a "script" and defines herbs as "little units of concentrated energy that nourish and energize the body and provide missing nutrients that supply the raw materials that we so desperately need to allow the body to do its job." The Herbal Hour instructions advise: "Tell your group that you are not there to prescribe or diagnose, that you are not a doctor so it is not legal for you to go beyond sharing information with your friends and neighbors. We like to explain, however, that it is their legal right to prescribe for themselves, so if they choose to use the information for themselves, they may do so."

"Sometimes," said Molly, "the medical field is not trained to know all the things that are beneficial to you. So that's why you're training yourself; you're learning on your own." When a distributor asked the difference between prescribing and recommending, Molly replied:

> It's just semantics. . . . Prescribing is actually saying: "If you have a cold, you need to take this common cold product that Nature's

Sunshine sells." That's prescribing. [You are recommending] if you say: "If I had a cold, I would want to take this product that would help my system. It would help me get rid of the cold." And so you're recommending then, using yourself as an example: "I would take this because I know it helps clean the mucus out of my system, and that will make the cold go away." So, knowing that, you can recommend what you would want to take for your cold. But saying, "For your cold, you need this product," is a prescription. Okay. So it's just a matter of semantics.

Then she proposed a similar alternative to diagnosis:

Somebody comes in, they're sneezing and running at the nose. If you say—"Oh, you have a cold. Here's a product for you."—that's diagnosing: You're telling them they have a cold, and you're not a doctor to tell them that. [But you could] say: "Well, from, you know, from what it looks like—it looks like, you know . . . you're having some respiratory troubles, and these are good respiratory disease products . . . probably the ones that you're thinking of."

Molly described these methods as "totally safe." Nevertheless, one distributor raised the question of lawsuits. Molly conceded that there had been cases involving distributors who "would not watch how they're recommending products." But she added:

It's not something you need to be concerned with . . . if you're just recommending the product and selling them. . . . There have been bills that have been tried to be passed in Congress . . . to limit what you can do, but those bills were not passed. And so anytime you're aware of any of these bills going on, you'll want to be in support of them not going through.

"We're not doing anything illegal or really weird," Molly assured us.

The Name Game

Next, Molly discussed NSP's "key products." She asked if anyone had had good results using any of the products for gastric ulcers. One distributor stated she advised people against drinking water with meals because it interferes with the action of hydrochloric acid and digestive enzymes. She said that drinking water with meals had been described to her as "the work of the devil." Another distributor concurred. "But," she added, "there are medical-nutritional doctors who say that's nonsense."

"It just shows you," Molly rejoined, "the different type of training that they have." But the distributor countered that the doctor to whom she had alluded was a "natural doctor"—a "nutritional" doctor. Molly responded that in nutrition schools, "nutritional philosophy is taught right along with the medical philosophy." Such schools, she claimed, teach that "if you do certain things in a certain way, then you don't need to be aware of any of these other things." She invited comments.

A distributor who later identified himself to me as a medical doctor trained in India responded that water taken with meals "basically doesn't affect the enzymes." But he added momentarily:

> If you're looking at [it from] your Western point of view, then the ["nutritional"] doctor will be right. If you're looking at [it from] a holistic point of view, then the quart of water will quench the fire, in . . . yin-yang [fashion]. . . . So it depends on who the guru is.

Later, in the dining room, this physician said he utilized Ayurvedic medicine, applied kinesiology ("muscle-testing"), and iridology in his practice. He further stated that he prescribed mostly herbs rather than pharmaceuticals, and excused NSP on the presumption that such organizations contribute to a much-needed overhaul of the medical establishment.

"A lot of these products you'll just take the rest of your life," said Molly, "because [of] the imbalance of your body, or you may have an inherently weakened state that you have to work with always." She indicated that the names of the herbal combination products refer to the conditions or organs they are designed to treat. For example, *U* stands for "ulcer"; *UC3-J*, for "ulcers, colitis, Crohn's disease, and celiac disease"; *AG-C* and *AG-X*, for "anti-gas"; and *BLG-X* for "bile, liver, and gallbladder." The letter "C," if it follows the hyphen, designates that the product is based on a traditional Chinese formula. Other letters following the hyphen refer to the designers of the formulas. For example, "A" refers to Paavo Airola and "X" refers to herbalist John R. Christopher (both of whom were naturopaths).

Molly claimed that, ideally, one should have three bowel movements daily, and declared that "everyone has a certain degree of parasites." She asked us how "optimal and proper elimination" can be supported. One distributor suggested *LBS II*, a "lower bowel stimulant" composed of nine herbs including cascara sagrada. Another described what happened as a result of her neglecting to tell one of her clients to ingest ample fluids with the herbal supplements he had been taking to "cleanse" himself:

> Totally unbeknownst to me, he was not drinking any water. He prided himself on being able to get by with only two glasses of fluid

a day. . . . And so he had horrendous stomach pains, and it wasn't until we went through everything [that we realized what the problem was]—and then he just went: "Oh, you mean you have to drink water?"

The audience laughed. "Horrible stomach pains," she emphasized. "I mean horrible. . . . I was just amazed that he didn't put that together at all . . . and I didn't even ask."

Another distributor acknowledged that she hadn't felt well during an herbal "cleanse." Molly attributed this feeling to the excretion of "toxins." "A lot of times when toxins are coming out of the body," she explained, "you experience the symptoms. That's the body's way of healing itself. So if you get a flu-like symptom with that cleanse, don't be alarmed." Molly referred to this reaction as a "healing crisis."

The Bottom Line

Nature's Sunshine is marketing hundreds of dubious products intended for the treatment of health problems. Its distributors are using unscientific methods as a basis for recommending products. The company also provides an extensive framework of false, misleading, and unproven statements with which to promote its products. I believe that, despite its elaborate system of disclaimers, NSP is breaking the law and encouraging its distributors to do so as well.

12

Nutripathy: Theologic Nutrition or Yellow Snow Job?

A "Unique Opportunity" to Improve Mankind?

I became aware of nutripathy through the tenth edition of *Bear's Guide to Earning Non-Traditional College Degrees* (1988), which lists the American College of Nutripathy (ACN) in Scottsdale, Arizona, as a "health-related school." The book describes it as a "nonresident" institution, founded in 1976, that offers "a practical (as contrasted with theoretical) approach to the healing of body, mind, and spirit" and awards bachelor's, master's, and doctoral degrees. It identifies the school's accrediting agency—the International Accrediting Commission for Schools, Colleges and Theological Seminaries—as "unrecognized." In response to my request for information in October 1989, the school mailed me a pamphlet entitled "Become a Nutripathic Practitioner," which included a sample of course topics and an order form for a $20 "student packet." The pamphlet states that the prospective student "may enroll in our off-campus division" and now has "a unique opportunity" to improve himself—"and, as a result, mankind."

All This and "Much More" for Just . . . ?

According to the nutripathy pamphlet:

American College of Nutripathy teaches you how to analyze your urine and saliva to analyze and remedy conditions of the body,

181

mind and spirit. You measure your urine and saliva to determine the frequency of your physical mechanism, mental consciousness, and spiritual awareness, resulting in an objective measurement of your wave pattern being emitted into the universe. Once this frequency is known, the wellness state (body-mind-spirit), including the immune system, can be analyzed and all problems rectified through natural, supportive means.

The course topics listed in the pamphlet included Bach flower remedies, colon therapy, color therapy, hair analysis, homeopathy, iridology, magnetic therapy, meditation and prayer, nutripathic food combining, radiesthesia, "rayid," reflexology, sclerology—"plus, much more!!!" "These curriculums," the pamphlet states, "will provide the knowledge and tools needed to objectively determine and correct nutritional imbalances, thereby eliminating the guesswork in nutritional support." It said of nutripathic food combining: "Proper food combining is a wonderful thing for many people, but some people just cannot handle eating in this manner." Program costs were not provided in the packet.

"You Have Been Directed to Us"

In November 1989, I mailed $20 to the school for its student packet. This included a forty-two-page curriculum guide and two books by school administrator Gary A. Martin, D.N, Ph.D., Th.D.: the tenth edition of *Nutripathy . . . The Final Solution to Your Health Dilemma* (1978) and *Don't Eat the Yellow Snow: A New Holistic Approach to Health.*

In the curriculum guide, a letter addressing the prospective student as "Dear Seeker" reiterates the "body-mind-spirit" message of the introductory pamphlet and describes nutripathy as "a fascinating development in the field of health and human consciousness"—"a revolutionary approach"—the way to finding one's "True Self"—indeed, "the study of the eternal way"! According to the guide, nutripathy views "the universe as the pulpit," "mankind as the congregation" and "life as a classroom." "You have been directed to us," the prospective student is told. "We have much work to do together. . . . You are at the right place at the right time."

A detailed outline of each of the three curricula cited in the introductory pamphlet is provided in the guide. The maximum time allowed for completion of any curriculum is twelve months. A high school diploma or equivalent is required for admission to the Basic Nutripathy curriculum. This curriculum covers such subjects as the spiritual significance of food, communication with God, cruel people, being upset, heavenly treasure, the Ten Commandments, "vital elements" in food, the answer to food faddism, the "Divine Diet," discovering a woman's mind, Kneipp leg baths, the "shocking truth" about prosperity, indebtedness, how to attract romance, the danger of gossip, the "magic power" of sex, and aspects of God.

The Basic Nutripathy Certificate, awarded upon completion of the first curriculum, is the prerequisite for admission to the Advanced Nutripathy curriculum. The latter includes such subjects as iridology, minerals, the "vital types" of man, a "vital" course on foods, sex-role development and self-concept, cardiac arrhythmia, crib death, masculine men, the end of the honeymoon, the incredible homemaker, the unforgettable woman, the origin of homosexuality in the home, "meridian imbalances," cancer, "advanced" cancer, "advanced true" cancer, "Doctor Death," seductive situations, physiognomy, reflexology, prolonged fasts for chronic ailments, behavioral kinesiology, "life energy," the "life" in food, how to "flow with the universe," genotypes, radiesthesia and radionics, chromotherapy, homeopathy, and accounting.

The Advanced Nutripathy Certificate is required for admission to the Nutripathic Practitioner curriculum, which covers such topics as: biochemistry, a reminder for the advanced soul, the power of prayer, orotate research, herb classifications, bowel problems, diabetes, "psycho-nutrition," "psycho-dietetics," heart disease, high blood pressure, food as one's best medicine, "contact healing," arthritis, how to remove emotional scars, prostate problems, impotence and frigidity, Easter Sunday, salvation, the "lost art" of Jesus, women's responsibilities, "natural/spiritual" man, accepting one's righteousness, kidney disease, alcoholism, schizophrenia, "The Tao of Physics," "The Way of Physics," diet and religion, real estate, tax write-offs, and Natural Hygiene.

If paid in advance, according to the guide, tuition costs $995 per curriculum. The guide states: "No refunds on materials received." In the guide I received in 1989, nine "educational tools" were recommended, including four videotape sets costing $400 each and a lab manual costing $1,000. The "degrees" offered in the 1989 guide include the baccalaureate, the master's degree, and doctorates in nutripathy (D.N.), philosophy (Ph.D.), and theology (Th.D.). But the guide also stated that the school's curricula were "accepted for full credit" toward "earned, accredited" bachelor's, master's, and Ph.D. degrees in "holistic science" by the International Institute of Holistic Sciences in Glendale, Arizona, at an additional cost of about $100 per degree. There has been no telephone listing in Glendale, Arizona, for this "institute" since I received the student packet, and it is not listed in either the tenth or eleventh edition of *Bear's Guide*.

The designation "D.N.," incidentally, also stands for "Doctor of Naprapathy," a credential conferred by the unaccredited Chicago National College of Naprapathy. This is a fringe school that offers training in "specific connective tissue manipulative therapy to relieve neurovascular interference, which may generate circulatory congestion and nerve irritation." Naprapathic practice includes nutritional counseling. Practitioners are not licensed.

A Blizzard of "Credentials"

On September 14, 1992, I called ACN. The woman who answered the phone said her name was Geneva. She informed me that the school had moved to larger quarters. I inquired about doctorates and accreditation. Geneva seemed not to recognize the name "International Institute of Holistic Sciences," but stated that ACN was no longer affiliated with Lafayette University. She told me that although ACN is not accredited, an accredited institution called North American University would accept all but nine credits toward a degree, and that these nine credits could be earned on a nonresident basis. North American University does have a telephone listing in Scottsdale, but when I called the "university," the phone was answered: "HealthWatchers." I requested information about accreditation, and was transferred to none other than Geneva, who explained that ACN and North American University were sharing offices.

A few days later I received an updated curriculum guide. In addition to the curricula described above, the new guide offers separate training and certification in "Biological Immunity Analysis" to "those who want to get involved in a practice immediately." It indicates that, depending upon which ACN curriculum the student has completed, a bachelor's, master's, or Doctor of Science degree can be obtained from Lafayette University in Aurora, Colorado, after completing nine additional credits at the "university." The mailing included a business-reply flyer for the Biological Immunity Research Institute in Scottsdale, Arizona. The flyer describes North American University's "off-campus" study program and lists thirty-five bachelor's, master's, and doctoral degrees obtainable from the "university."

Lafayette University was part of a "paper conglomerate" that began in Indiana in 1983 as the American Nutritional Medical Association

(ANMA), moved to Colorado in 1987, and evolved into the American Nutrimedical Association and International Alliance of Nutrimedical Associations. Initially, ANMA operated John F. Kennedy College of Nutrimedical Arts and Sciences (American Nutrimedical University), which offered correspondence courses leading to "degrees," "diplomas," or certificates in "nutritional medicine," "chiropathic medicine," "neuroreflex therapy," "naturodermatology," homeopathy, hypnotherapy, and "nutrimedical" counseling. "Board certification" was also available in a variety of medically unrecognized specialties.

ANMA also offered a Doctor of Nutritional Medicine (N.M.D.) "degree," which could be obtained by taking a correspondence course for $1,895 or—for those who had a suitable doctoral degree or qualifying experience—by filling out an application and paying $250. When ANMA moved to Colorado, holders of an NMD diploma were invited to exchange it for one from Lafayette University. The 1991 ANMA directory lists eighty-three members in the United States. Gary Martin, NMD, was listed in several previous editions.

A 1990 Lafayette University flyer offered resident and external programs in wellness sciences, botanical sciences, conservation and natural sciences, and eleven subjects related to pastoral counseling, theology, or other religious matters. In September 1992, however, there was no telephone listing for "Lafayette University" in Aurora, Colorado, and my calls to the phone numbers in its flyer and on its letterhead proved fruitless.

"God, the Vital Force within You"

In the introduction to *Nutripathy . . . The Final Solution*, Gary Martin defines nutripathy as "the latest concept in nutrition. . . . a science of health using specific nutritional techniques." Yet he hastens to add that "Nutripaths DO NOT treat anything," and that "Nutripathy has NOTHING to do with disease." Citing *Webster's* definition of "doctor," Martin defines the "Doctor of Nutripathy" as "a learned and authoritative teacher of sound nutrition." He claims that nutripaths satisfy "a great need in the practice of an already licensed doctor" because "many doctors are too busy to take the time required to counsel you concerning your nutritional needs." Martin further states:

> Nutripathy is based upon the religious concept that God created man with certain nutritional requirements and placed the source of

those dietary requirements in natural foods. Nutripaths believe that a properly combined diet of natural foods will allow a person to live in a state of perfect health.

Martin also claims that "many 'diseases' are not diseases at all, but merely the result of nutritional deficiencies, which result in cellular contamination, which is the end product of improper diet." In Chapter 1, he explains that the nutripath cannot legally "mention nor concern themself" with disease, yet he describes this fact as "amazing." He adds that even if nutripaths could focus on disease, "they would realize that the cause of most health problems is nutritional in nature anyway." If "you still feel badly" after visiting many doctors, says Martin, "you probably have been talking to the wrong people." "Many times," he claims, "mysterious conditions defying medical diagnosis and treatment turn out to be simple nutritional problems." He states that the reader "may be able to gain a whole new life of good health" by visiting a nutripath. Martin calls orthodox nutrition "a shotgun approach based upon educated guesswork," as contrasted with the nutripathic nutritional program, which he says is tailored to one's specific needs.

Chapter 1 also features the story of nutripathy's origin: As a student at a chiropractic college, Martin became progressively "aware that nutrition as well as proper nerve energy reaching the body's millions of cells was the answer to obtaining and keeping perfect health." In 1976, he met a biochemist specializing in agricultural nutrition who was "convinced that the same testing methods used by farmers to produce healthy plants by altering the condition of the soil could be applied to human urine and saliva to develop a picture of that person's nutritional deficiencies." But the biochemist was "poisoned" by the establishment and "incapacitated" for about a year, and so Martin was "forced" to continue his nutrition education through the "school of hard knocks." The concept of nutripathy finally came in answer to his prayers—"the divine idea. . . . definitely a gift from God." Martin then expresses his belief in creationism: "Man is not the evolutionary product of an amoeba" but "was created by God, in the image of God." Citing *Genesis,* he states that all requirements for life, except water, are found in fruits, nuts, seeds, and vegetables "as nature provided them." Common sense, he writes, "tells us that God created foods just the way God wanted them."

Chapter 2 of Martin's book refers to pioneer Natural Hygienists Sylvester Graham, Russell Thacker Trall, and John Tilden, and to Max Gerson and Gerson therapy. All of these men, according to Martin, shared a belief in "toxemia. . . . the concept that health problems develop only when the body becomes loaded down with 'garbage' and after being deprived of proper nutrition."

Chapter 3, entitled "You, the Pawn," begins with an attack on the pharmaceutical industry, the American Medical Association, the Food and Drug Administration, the U.S. Post Office, and the Internal Revenue Service. Martin asserts that one must be "born again"—"nutritionally speaking"—in order to "break loose from the grip" of the "giant corporations." "Choose to be born again," he exhorts the reader. "Experience a life without doctors and hospitals." Martin interprets a saying attributed to Christ—"Ye cannot serve God and mammon"—to mean that "you will ultimately have to choose between commercially prepared foods and your health." Citing *Corinthians*, he states:

Man is the temple [of God], and you should not defile that temple; you should not eat, drink or apply anything to your body which destroys, even if little by little, that magnificent temple. If you do, you must expect to reap what you sow.

In Chapter 4, Martin explains that nutripaths test urine, saliva, and hair because they are obtained easily. "The urine," he writes, "is a good end result representation of the nutritional reactions of your body." But nutripaths do not test feces because they "are largely undigested food particles and do not have that much to do with waste matter resulting from cell metabolism." Nutripaths test urine and saliva for several "components"—sugar, pH, electrolytes, albumin ("urine debris"), nitrates, and ammonia—whose significance is explained in Chapters 5 to 10 of his book. The Nutripathic Questionnaire for patients includes questions about prescription medications and recent surgery, but Martin advises prospective clients to ask the nutripath only one question about drugs: "Do you have a *Physician's Desk Reference*, and, if so, would you please copy what it has to say regarding my drugs?" The *PDR*, says Martin, contains "terrible information."

"Drugs are a fraud!" declares Martin in Chapter 12. "All healing has always been, is, and will always remain the exclusive province of God, the vital Force within you." In a later chapter, he writes:

If you do not believe in God, and in man as God's creation, then you probably won't believe in the specific dietary needs decreed by God. If this is the case, then you should consider NOT going to see a Nutripath. Chances are your faith is not strong enough to withstand the detoxification process.

In Chapter 19, Martin states: "You may not know of a Nutripath near you. There may not be enough of them for the telephone company to have created a separate category for them." He invites the reader unable to find a nutripath to request such information from ACN, which charges $20 "to pay for the computer search."

How to Become a "Perfected Master"

The "Notice and Disclaimer" in *Don't Eat the Yellow Snow* identifies its target audience as "the professional Health Practitioner who has an interest in holistic concepts." It concedes that "the concepts presented herein may be considered by some to be controversial and unorthodox, and cannot, at this time, be proven in such a manner that will satisfy medical science." Yet it describes the material as "the result of over twelve years of extensive research, study and practical experience." "I am convinced," writes Martin, "that there is a scientific and mathematical relationship—a cause and effect—between certain shifts in the body chemistry and the eventual outbreak of disease." He claims:

> I have learned how to make a biochemical analysis of the urine and saliva . . . and, from that analysis, develop a profile. . . . From that profile, with certain higher mathematical calculations, it is possible to determine the nature and meridian location of any imbalance affecting the person. Any person having the same profile would have the same imbalance. It is not necessary to rely on symptoms related to the doctor by the patient. It is also possible to develop a psychological profile.

Martin's urine/saliva test and his "Nutripathic Profile" are based on the work of Cary Reams, a self-proclaimed biophysicist who developed the test over fifty years ago and was prosecuted in the 1970s for practicing medicine without a license. Reams, too, claimed that his work was divinely inspired. The perfect Nutripathic Profile, according to Martin, "portrays MINIMUM RESISTANCE to God's Universal Laws." This apparently refers to the degree of resistance necessary for optimal health. Martin adds: "It also represents minimum resistance present in the mind, which means the person with the perfect profile is living in accordance with Universal Principle." Such a person, he states, "is well on the way to becoming a perfected Master, which is everyone's purpose for existing." The perfect profile looks like this:

1.5   6.4/6.4   7   1   3/3

The first number, 1.5, refers to the level of sugar in the urine; 6.4 refers to the pH of urine and saliva, respectively; 7, to the level of electrolytes in the urine; 1, to the amount of albumin ("cell debris") in the urine; and 3, to the respective amounts of nitrates and ammonia in the urine. The first half of the profile (1.5, 6.4/6.4 and 7) is said to be an expression of "energy input" and to bear on digestive and metabolic "efficiency." The second half (7, 1, and 3/3) "tells how much energy your metabolism is using." As these numbers "travel away from normal," Martin explains, they indicate that more energy is consumed to support the metabolic functions of the body. Martin states that "low energy input" and "high energy drain" may add up to "degeneration, rot, decay and death." Examples are given of profiles purported to indicate an excess of "what if," resentment, impatience, fear, and intenseness ("spiritual concentration").

The Enterprising Pastor

Martin also heads: the Eternal Life Center, a nondenominational church; Nutripathic Formulas, Inc., a for-profit company that sells nutritional supplements and various other health-related items by mail; and Natural Health Outreach, a clinic that offers counseling on-site or by mail. He is founder and pastor of the church, of which his school is a tax-exempt "educational ministry," and has identified the degrees conferred by the school as "religious degrees, used solely for religious purposes within a religious organization" [*Nutrition Forum,* September 1987].

Nutripathic Formulas has marketed well over five hundred products. Nearly 350 are now sold under the trademark "HealthWatchers System." These include a "transmutation plaque" costing about $53; *Toxoid Formula* and *Toxoid* crystals, moisturizer, lotion, ointment, shampoo, and hair conditioner; herbal, homeopathic, and oral glandular preparations; vitamin and mineral supplements; a hair analysis kit for pets; and many books, brochures, and audiovisuals dealing with nutripathic methods and wares.

Nutripathic Formulas distributes a free newsletter called *HealthWatchers Handbook,* which announces newly available products, associates products with various health problems, and includes testimonials. The November/December issue announced a two-week "retreat program" that included "testing, counseling, diet, detoxing, chiropractic, colonics, massage, reflexology, stress processing, and more." The 1992 *HealthWatchers* catalog includes a "symptomatology/usage" index, which associates products with diseases, symptoms, and other conditions, and with bodily parts and processes. Conditions include air pollution, aloofness, ambition, compulsiveness, courage, frustration, and homosexuality. The catalog's description of *Toxoid Formula* is:

> A negatively ionized, specially prepared solution of minerals well known for their healing properties. . . . just a catalyst to help the body do its thing more effectively. . . . Drink it. Spray it on and rub it in. . . . We use it for adhesions, arthritis, colitis, diverticulitis, wounds, scar tissue, moles, skin problems, rashes, inflammations, sore throats, surgery, warts, ulcers, burns and more!

A flyer claims that *Toxoid Formula* "stimulates the production of antibodies on the body tissue surface." The flyer concedes that the mechanism of action is unknown. "However," it states, "we do know that it *does work.* The special process used to allow the natural crystalline formation and bonding of the minerals used in this formulation account for its effectiveness." *Toxoid Formula* is recommended in the flyer for "any condition ending in 'itis' or 'osis'"—but this recommendation is attributed to an unnamed young lady from Indiana. The flyer itself states: "WE MAKE NO MEDICINAL CLAIMS for this product. The TESTIMONI-ALS which are reproduced in this brochure are furnished for educational purposes only."

Another *HealthWatchers* product is *Ultra Vita Florum*, an "en-hanced" version of *Vita Florum*. The 1992 catalog describes the latter as a "unique spiritual healing agent from England." A 1989 issue of the clinic's newsletter quotes an unnamed British doctor as stating it has "the potential to heal everybody and everything." It adds:

> Many users claim "it can and does heal just about anything in the body, mind and spirit, from accidents to chronic disorders." Unlike certain remedies, it requires no diagnosis, since it consists of one single preparation in many forms (water, tablets, lotion, ointment, salve, foliar spray, talcum). VITA FLORUM constitutes a su-premely simple self-therapy for every type of illness or shortcom-ing or inability to cope.

A brochure explains that "VITA FLORUM has been energized with HOMEOVITIC TRANSCREATIONAL energy by Elizabeth Bellhouse. This is a spiritual, not a physical process. It has spiritual properties only." The newsletter presents before-and-after Kirlian photographs as "dramatic evidence of healing energy at work."

Following the "cover story" on *Vita Florum* is a case study of a ten-year-old student named Barbara whose "presenting problem" was inability to walk without crutches. According to the article, there was "no medical explanation for this disability." The child was a client of a "successful" nutripath who "does not have electricity because of religious reasons." Nutripathic analysis of her urine revealed an electrolyte deficiency. The article explains:

> When electrolytes are low in the urine we can expect an alkaline blood [and].... *poor nerve energy transmission between the brain and muscles.* Acid is where we get energy. The reason normal blood is alkaline (7.46) is because the cells are using the acid. Barbara is not delivering acid to her cells. They have no energy. *No wonder she is on crutches without the ability to walk.*

The article states, however, that thanks to the Nutripathic Program, Barbara "is now running and playing like a normal child."

"Martin Is Making Us All Look Like Quacks"

In 1987, *Nutrition Forum* published an article by reporter Jeff South, who quoted Gary Martin's evaluation of a client: "The man may be in the early stages of slowly turning into a garbage dump, rotting from the inside, thereby experiencing nothing more at this time than an extreme energy loss." The article noted that naturopathic officials in Arizona had called ACN's curriculum a sham and that a member of the Arizona Naturopathic Physicians Board of Examiners had stated: "Martin is making us all look like quacks." In 1985 the board condemned the college as an "imminent danger to the health and well-being of the citizens of the state," and asked the U.S. Postal Service to shut down the school. A naturopath in Phoenix turned various school publications over to the authorities and concluded: "Gary Martin is creating a nationwide network of unqualified 'doctors' who know a lot more about lining their pockets than they do about healing." In the same year, under a new state law, the Arizona Board for Private Postsecondary Education began regulating private degree-granting institutions, and a panel advised Martin that he would need a license for his school. According to the board's minutes, Martin refused to apply for a license or to obey a subpoena to appear before the panel. Instead, he initiated a lawsuit against the board later that year, which was dropped when both parties agreed to attempt a resolution. Arizona law exempts from its definition of the practice of medicine "any person while engaged in the practice of religion, treatment by prayer, or the laying on of hands as a religious rite or ordinance."

In New York, ACN graduate Marcos Freddy Martinez pleaded guilty in 1987 to practicing medicine without a license and received a year's probation. Nevertheless, "Doctor of Nutripathy" and "Biological Systems Analyst" Michael Biamonte has advertised "the most complete nutritional analysis available" in the Health Services section of New York's *Free Spirit Magazine*. In a similar periodical, *Newlife,* a classified ad describes him as a "Certified Clinical Nutritionist" (C.C.N.) and a naturopath, which is defined as "one who uses only safe, natural approaches." Another East Coast nutripath I know of not only practiced her chosen profession, but also wrote local newspaper columns, some of which identified her as "Dr." without indicating the dubious nature of her "degree."

The Bottom Line

The American College of Nutripathy has granted hundreds of "degrees" to people throughout the United States and abroad. Its teachings do not correspond to accepted biological, nutritional, and medical facts. The harm caused by its graduates cannot be measured, but it is difficult to imagine their rendering any worthwhile service as "health professionals."

Federal laws require that products marketed for the prevention or treatment of disease be safe, effective, and adequately labeled for their intended uses. Gary Martin's marketing of *Toxoid Formula* and *Ultra Vita Florum* appears to be violating these provisions. Despite disclaimers, he and some of his "graduates" appear to have been practicing medicine without a license.

13

Mail-Order Nutrition:
Journey into Mystery

"Elvis & his mom were lovers!"

"Frisco woman spends $51,000 on plastic surgery to change herself into a Japanese!"

"Insurance Company Replaces Kidnapped Children with Brand-New Kids!"

"Newlyweds take granny's corpse on their honeymoon!"

With headlines like these distracting me, it is perhaps a wonder that I ever completed this project—a survey of ninety-four popular magazines and newspapers ranging from the immediately recognizable to the quite obscure. I examined at least one issue of each periodical, for a total of 134 issues. My goal was to delineate the nature and prevalence of advertisements for nutrition-related products available by mail. I limited the survey to early 1992 issues of lay periodicals containing at least one article pertaining to human health or health care. All ads included in the database promoted products intended primarily for human consumption. It did not include ads for books, "skin-nourishing" cosmetics, or herbal preparations for which no nutrition-related claims were made. Some of the advertised products turned out to be unavailable directly from the advertiser but are obtainable from "health food" stores or discount mail-order houses.

Mysterious and Dubious Products

In thirty-three (5 percent) of the 612 ads noted, it is not entirely clear whether the product is ingestible. Where suitability for ingestion was

193

obscure or negated, the ad was excluded from the database. For example, a classified ad in *The Advocate*, a gay paper, reads:

AIDS—CANCER—ETC. This off the shelf product can possibly be the cure. Astounding information, send $10.00 to H.O.P.E.

An ad for an ingestible product was likewise excluded if nutritional relevance was obscure or negated, unless the product was claimed to facilitate muscular hypertrophy. In *To Your Health*, a classified ad for an unnamed product said to be "doctor recommended" bids: "Repair your villi and regain your health." In the *National Enquirer*, an ad for *The Energy Pill*, an herbal preparation, makes no nutrition-related claims, but promises a "*safe* and *reliable*" increase in vigor and acuity. A classified ad in the *National Examiner* proffers tapes at $12 apiece:

LOSE WEIGHT while you sleep! Easy, safe, effective. No diet, no pills. Change your eating habits, improve your life overnight.

Another proffers a "scientific secret" for burning fat without exercise or drugs, discoverable via a "900" number at a cost of $2 per minute. Yet another, in the tabloid *News Extra*, offers a chart and booklet "formulated by well renowned Dr. Nutrit." A classified ad in *New Frontier* reads:

SELF-PURIFICATION THERAPY. No-nonsense herbal cleansing program safely removes 35 feet of old, toxic matter from the entire digestive tract in seven days. Old fears are released, leaving one feeling liberated on all levels.

The reader is asked to mail $2 for a seventeen-page information packet. Very similar ads in *East West Natural Health* and *New Age Journal* indicate that from twenty to forty feet of this matter can be removed, and request $3 for a ten-page information packet. I suppose that seventeen pages and a sure thirty-five feet constitute a better buy, but perhaps I am quibbling.

Nearly half (305) of the ads included in the database make claims related to health or to bodybuilding. Over 17 percent (108) of all the ads make specific claims, and at least 5 percent (33) allude to paranormal concepts. (For the purposes of this study I did not consider homeopathic products "paranormal," even though homeopathy is a vitalistic system.)

Placebos

Placebos are substances that have no specific physiological effect on the body. I can think of no better example of an ingestible placebo than

Tachyon Water. "Tachyon" is a term in physics for a particle hypothesized to travel faster than light and backward in time. Experiments attempting to detect such particles have proved unpromising, however, and nearly all physicists doubt their existence. Yet Tachyon Energy Research in Beverly Hills, California, advertises a variety of "tachyon" items in *Newlife*, including beads, neckties, and mineral water. The company defines tachyon energy as a "life-force," a "subtle energy," and a "spiritual quality," which is faster-than-light and omnipresent. It claims that scientists in Japan have developed products "uniquely processed to focus this life-force." How was this done? The mailing I received from the company included two reprints from *Raum & Zeit*, a periodical focused on "alternative methods of medicine and physics." One article describes the means of extraction as "the inventor's secret." A flier lists six dysfunctions treated with tachyon energy: allergies, bronchitis, cystic mastitis, knee injuries, cervical and

Table 13-1. Placebos

Product/Price	Description	Claims and Comments
Tachyon 21 About $40.00 for 2- to 3-month supply	Mineral water infused with universal "life-force"	Restores and increases energy and vitality; enhances natural defense mechanisms; organizes the Life Force; an antidote to pollution; can help conquer subclinical illness
Stop Drops $34.95 for 1-month supply	Homeopathic preparation	Curbs appetite and craving for sugar
Oscillococcinum $2.00 per dose	Homeopathic preparation	"Natural relief from symptoms of flu" [The ad refers to chicken soup, which is a better bet.]
Testosterone 6X $24.95 for 1-month supply	Homeopathic preparation	Helps users "get big" and increases the "aggressiveness" of workouts; outperforms anything legal
Testosterone $30.00 for 40-day supply	Homeopathic preparation	Increases strength and muscle mass
Starlight Elixirs $10.95 per ounce	"Made from the light of individual stars and planets"	"Will assist in the evolution of your physical, mental, emotional, and spiritual selves"

lumbar spinal sprains, and "mild large intestine dysbiosi." An accompanying handwritten letter stated:

> I sincerely believe that this revolutionary technology will be a boon to mankind and our hopes and desires are to promote a healthier and happier lifestyle—a change that is badly needed, not only here in America, but all over the world.

Tachyon Energy Research apparently markets aggressively: After I left my number on the company's answering device, a representative phoned me several times from California, once after 7 P.M. EDT on Independence Day (a Saturday).

In the same issue of *Newlife*, naturopath David Blodgett offers his own testimonial on tachyon energy and writes: "The tachyon seems to act as a catalyst and balance for the life energy and healing process, with no side effects or contra-indications." He concludes: "The time has finally come when we can begin to replace drugs with energy for healing."

Homeopathic preparations are another example of placebos. Homeopathy is based on the utterly nonsensical idea that a vast assortment of substances can have powerful therapeutic effects on the body when administered in infinitesimal amounts—indeed, even if not a molecule of the substance is present in the preparation. A classified ad in *Health World* reads: "Homeopathy for Weight Loss! Average weight loss: 18–22 lbs. in first month. STOP DROPS curb your appetite and sugar cravings naturally." One exhibitor at a 1991 symposium sponsored by the Foundation for the Advancement of Innovative Medicine (FAIM) marketed "the new, improved" version of this product, describing it as an all-natural, fast-acting, fabulous alternative to the "old" way to lose weight. The "old" way, according to the company, consists of a "strict diet-exercise program. . . . demanding, tough, restrictive and frankly boring."

Oscillococcinum is another homeopathic product. Readers of the *New Age Journal* and *The 1992 New Age Sourcebook* are asked to think of it "like chicken soup when you're coming down with the flu!" Doing so just *might*, via a placebo effect, render the product beneficial.

Testosterone 6X "Out Performs Anything Legal," according to a display in *MuscleMag International*. The shapely model pictured in the ad says it's "just the product you've been looking for to help you get the body that men respect and drives women like me crazy." But *Testosterone 6X* is a homeopathic product. Thus, if it does help users "get big" and increase the "aggressiveness" of their workouts, as the ad claims, it does so via the placebo effect. The designation "6X" refers to the homeopathic "potency" of 1 part per million, an amount of testosterone too small to produce any significant physical or mental change.

"Wonder Foods"

"Food" may be defined as any substance that contains at least one absorbable nutrient and can appease hunger or thirst. Thus, royal jelly, spirulina, and wheat grass are foods, and advertisements calling them so may evoke a sense of safety. Over-the-counter nutritional supplements, including herbal preparations represented as such, are generally regulated as foods if they are marketed without claims on their label. However, these products are legally transformed into drugs when accompanied by claims

Table 13-2. "Wonder Foods"

Product/Price	Description	Claims and Comments
Foodform Manna	"Whole food concentrate"	Directly nourishes every cell in the body
MegaFood About $11.00 for 1-month supply	"Predigested" whole-food concentrates made with Saccharomyces pyrenoidsa, a single-celled plant	Over 1,000 times more potent than ordinary whole food. Absorption rate is up to 16 times that of "natural" vitamins. Plants add "Life Force" to vitamins and minerals via "miraculous Life/Growth Processes." Only MegaFood—which is grown, not manufactured—attains total harmony with your body through these processes. [Subjects in absorption studies were rats.]
Celtic Seasalt $12.00 per pound	"Contains 84 minerals that are appearently [sic] perfectly balanced for human nutrition"	Alone will maintain life, destroy toxins and detrimental bacteria, and enhance all organic functions; causes gray hair to return to normal color
Aloe vera beverage $17.81 for quart	Preservative-free "energy drink" containing 50% aloe vera juice, ascorbic acid, electrolytes, fructose, an herbal tea blend, natural apple flavor, "etc."	Relieves arthritis, diabetes, and high blood pressure

that they can prevent, cure, mitigate, or treat a disease.

Advertisers often engage in puffery to portray products as "wonder foods." For example, a display in *Vegetarian Times* calls *Foodform Manna* "the world's most nutritious whole food concentrate." According to the ad, vitamin supplements cannot help someone suffering from fatigue, irritability, and lowered resistance, "because even the so-called 'natural' ones have no food value." *Earth Source* and *MegaFood* are similarly promoted. *Earth Source* is said to provide "more than just natural vitamins and minerals. It provides the natural energy of over 65 wholesome food factors, including spirulina, chlorella, wheat grass juice and sprouted barley juice." *MegaFood* is "up to 16 times more effective than manufactured 'natural' vitamins," according to an ad in *The 1992 New Age Sourcebook*. The ad invites readers to call a toll-free number to obtain a free booklet. This, it says, "includes testimonials that claim dramatic health improvements using *MegaFood*." The alleged results include far fewer colds, stronger nails, shinier hair, rejuvenated sex life, and increased energy. Claims like these are illegal but seldom attract regulatory attention because they are considered relatively insignificant,

Advertising claims for *Flora Balance* are made via testimonials ascribed to unnamed individuals. Its active ingredients are not indicated. However, in a *Vegetarian Times* ad, a "Doctor of Oriental Medicine" describes the product as "the kind of food we need to help the immune system." In *For Women First*, a full-page ad from Bee-Alive, Inc., tells how royal jelly helped the company president and her son overcome chronic weakness and lethargy. The ad describes royal jelly as a "natural food" and a "wonderful, God-given substance." The facts are otherwise: scientific studies have found that royal jelly has no practical physiological effect in humans.

I also noted that many food products were promoted with adjectives that have little or no nutritional significance. These included: "adaptogenic whole foods," air-dried tomato slices, "all natural" pork, deli cheesecake, herbal tonic soups, nongelatin capsules, "organic" cherries, "organic" baked beans, unleavened bread, and whole-spelt flour.

"Supernutrients"

A full-page ad in several magazines for *MDR Fitness Tabs* asks: "What would you spend to feel energized, strengthen your immune system, revitalize skin, hair and nails, and improve your overall health?" "MDR" here stands for "Medical Doctors' Research," the product's manufacturer, not for "Minimum Daily Requirements," which are the outmoded forerunners of the RDAs (Recommended Dietary Allowances). The ad does not state explicitly that taking the product will affect any health problem. Rather, it asks loaded questions and alludes to supporting research. Nevertheless, any claim that a product strengthens the immune system is a "drug" claim and therefore illegal. Other companies evince less concern for the law. For example, a classified ad in *Newlife* for an aloe vera beverage (see table) claims that the product relieves arthritis, diabetes, and high blood pressure.

The term "nutrient" can refer to any food-related substance that can contribute significantly to the maintenance of life. "Essential nutrient" usually refers to any naturally occurring nutrient that is either not produced or insufficiently produced by the human body and whose presence in the body is essential for normal functioning. All vitamins and certain minerals and amino acids are essential nutrients.

In many people, the word "nutrient" evokes a sense not only of safety but of utility. Unfortunately, the health-food industry claims that some nonnutrients are nutrients, that some nonessential nutrients are essential, and that many questionable or worthless "dietary supplements" have therapeutic value. In my survey, for example, I noted a liquid mineral preparation called *Genesis 1000* advertised in *Health World* as "*the* oxygen supplement." The ad quotes a previous issue of *Health World*, which describes *Genesis 1000* as "the vital nutrient." In *Let's Live*, another display for the same product refers to oxygen as "vitamin O." Oxygen is neither a nutrient nor a vitamin.

Nutrionics in Concord, California, sent me a flyer describing the cofactors lipoic acid and coenzyme Q_{10} as "non-vitamin nutrients" that are "essential nonetheless." The flyer proceeds:

> Many scientific studies have shown that supplements of these non-vitamin nutrients may produce measurable benefits to our bodies, even though they are not vitamins or *dietarily* essential in the strictest sense. In other words, just because our bodies can make *some* CoQ_{10} or Lipoic Acid . . . from our normal diet, it does not automatically follow that our bodies will *always* make the *optimal* amounts needed to catalyze our cellular energy production cycles to provide all the energy we need in our lives.

The foregoing argument is gobbledygook designed to distract the reader from the relevant question of whether one's "non-vitamin nutrient" status is a reasonable concern or the stuff of hypochondria. Coenzyme Q_{10} (CoQ_{10} or ubidecorenone) is one of a class of chemical compounds called

Table 13-3. "Supernutrients"

Product/Price	Description	Claims and Comments
MDR Fitness Tabs $5.00 for 10-day trial supply	"A.M." and P.M." multivitamin formulas for men and women	Certain nutrients are best taken in the morning and others at night. Strengthens the immune system; revitalizes skin, hair, and nails; improves overall health; combats fatigue
Genesis 1000	Liquid mineral preparation called "oxygen supplement"	Has unique antiviral and antibacterial properties; free radical scavenger; improves stamina and endurance
Body Essential silica Gel $14.95 for 7 ounces	Silicon supplement	Helps smooth skin, add luster and sheen to hair, and harden nails; plays an important role in stopping the growth of malignant tumors
Thioctic (lipoic acid) $15.25 for 50 capsules Source Naturals CoQ10 (coenzyme Q10) $22.79 for 30 capsules	Cofactors ("non-vitamin nutrients")	"The Keys To Optimal Energy" (One's nonvitamin cofactor status is the stuff of hypochondria.

ubiquinones. The prefix "ubi," meaning "everywhere," refers to the wide distribution in nature of CoQ_{10} and its chemical relatives. CoQ_{10} is synthesized by body cells, where it participates in the conversion of nutrients into a storage form of chemical energy. Pharmaceutical CoQ_{10} may be a useful adjunct in the medical treatment of some cases of chronic heart failure, but "self-prescribed" CoQ_{10} supplements are unlikely to be effective.

A silicon supplement called *Body Essential silica Gel* is advertised in *New Age Journal*, *The 1992 New Age Sourcebook*, and *Let's Live* as needed "to help smooth skin, add luster and sheen to hair, and harden nails." The product is said to be derived from crystals, which "have long been thought to possess mysterious powers." NatureWorks of Agoura Hills, California, sent me a booklet about it and a flyer listing the "healing properties" of silica. The flyer states that the German county of Daun has the lowest cancer rate in western Europe and suggests that the rate is low because "the water from the spring contains an abundance of silica."

Table 13-4. "Diet Aids"

Product/Price	Description	Claims and Comments
Fat Busters $12.95 for 1-month supply	"Miracle herb"	Breaks the fat chain. "With these power pills there is no starvation or hunger, only boundless energy."
Mini White Cross $3/100 tablets Mini Pink Heart $4–$6 per 100	25 mg ephedrine, a decongestant and stimulant	Opens up the system. [Side effects include insomnia and nervousness.]
Large Pink Heart $4–$6 per 100	200 mg caffeine	Keeps you alert and active. [Not a genuine diet aid.]
Quick Loss $5.00 for 100 "time-released" caplets	75 mg phenyl-propanolamine (PPA), appetite suppressant	Strongest nonprescription diet aid available; can help decrease inches and pounds. Fine print states that a calorie-restricted diet must be followed. Doses high enough to suppress appetite may produce headaches, blurring of vision, nervousness, insomnia, dizziness, palpitations, and blood-pressure elevations.
Super Slim Diet Plan $19.95 for 60 tablets	Anti-Fat Wonder Weapon. Active ingredient not revealed in ad.	Dissolves and drains away years of excess, stubborn fat, flab, and fluids; then tightens, lifts, and firms your body. [The tablets are to be used as part of the diet plan, about which no specifics are provided.]
Safe herbal capsules $6.95 for "starter supply"	Amazing new product for guaranteed weight loss	Effects weight loss without exercise or dieting. [Ad reveals neither ingredients nor quantity of product.]
Nature's Cleanser	Herbal laxative	Controls weight immediately without calorie restriction or dietary change by eliminating waste such as fatty tissue, cellulite, toxins, mucus, hardened fecal matter, and harmful drug residues
Diet Pep $12.95 for 1-month supply	All-natural herbal supplement containing kola nut, ma huang, Siberian ginseng, pugongying, zingiber, kelp, passion flower, and Gymnema sylvestre	Curbs appetite, reduces desire for sweets, and provides energy needed for sticking to diet. [Ma huang contains ephedrine, a nasal decongestant that can elevate blood pressure and cause insomnia and nervousness. "Pugongying" is the Chinese word for dandelion, a common weed of no therapeutic value. The roots may stimulate the appetite slightly. "Zingiber" is a fancy name for ginger, a gastrointestinal irritant.]

"Diet Aids"

The word "drug" usually refers to any substance that can (or is claimed to) chemically alter at least one function of a living organism. In the 1940s, mail-order ads for *Kelpidine*—a dried seaweed product—pictured a shapely young woman in a bathing suit, and suggested that, by following the Kelpidine Reducing Plan, one could lose three to five pounds a week without exercise, "yet eat plenty." This plan's caloric allowance was between 800 and 1,200, a calorie intake low enough to cause weight loss with or without the *Kelpidine*. Ruses like this are still common, but not all obesity treatments are as harmless as *Kelpidine*.

"Diet Aids/Body Stimulants" reads one of the headings in the classified ad section of the *National Examiner*. One ad refers only to "WHITE CROSS, pink hearts." Toll-free phone calls brought flyers listing, among other products, tablets and capsules whose active ingredient is caffeine, ephedrine, or phenylpropanolamine (PPA). Ephedrine is a bronchodilator used to treat colds and asthma. Its actions are similar to those of adrenalin but last longer. Both ephedrine and PPA can suppress the appetite somewhat. Ephedrine *may* increase energy expenditure and metabolic rate. Its most common side effects are insomnia and nervousness, which are also side effects of PPA. (For persons so affected, the flyers also offer diphenhydramine tablets as a "sleep aid.") Doses of PPA high enough to suppress the appetite may also cause headaches, blurring of vision, dizziness, palpitations, and elevations in blood pressure. An ad in *Cosmopolitan* for *Mini Thins* (ephedrine) and *Mini Slims* (PPA) advises prospective buyers to consult their physician before using the products. This advice appears in small print, but should not be taken lightly. It would be better to avoid PPA diet products entirely. Although they may suppress appetite temporarily, they have not been proven effective for long-term weight control. Ironically, one company selling such drugs calls itself "Mother Natures."

Not all diet aids have a high-tech aura. More mundane but supposedly "revolutionary" nonetheless is a "diet bread" advertised in *Woman's Day*. "Just eat our high fiber bread with your food," the classified ad states, and watch the pounds melt away!

"Ergogenic Aids"

The term "ergogenic aid" refers to any procedure, device, or substance claimed to increase vitality, facilitate muscular hypertrophy, or improve the performance of a specific activity. Body By Jay Fitness Enterprises markets a variety of supplements to the "drug-free athlete." The company's display in *Men's Exercise* and *Natural Physique* begins by implying that users of its products will gain thirty pounds of "solid muscle" in four weeks. However, the text of the ad then hedges. "We don't claim miracles

Table 13-5. "Ergogenic Aids"

Product/Price	Description	Claims and Comments
Oxygen Cocktail	Oxygenated sports recovery drink, "The Soviet Athlete's Secret Weapon!"	Improves performance, increases endurance, and shortens recovery time
Body Amino Test R' Own 1000 $39.95 for 1- to 2-month supply	Herbal Anabolic Formula	Guarantees success in competing against others or building oneself. Scientifically tested and patented. [So what? Testing something and proving it are very different things. Proof of effectiveness is not required to obtain a patent.]
Ripped Fast $17.95 for 1-month supply	Ten-way lipotropic/ergogenic formula containing "near vitamins" choline and inositol, 2 mg vitamin B-6, betaine hydrochloride, two amino acids, beta-sitosterol [a plant compound], and three herbs: buchu leaves, hops, and uva ursi	"The Definitive Fat Burner" will get you "ripped"; puts you in contest shape all of the time; accelerates the fat-burning process; and advances the human form when used with any type of exercise program. ["Ripped," in physical culture lingo, means lean with large, well-defined muscles. Plant sterols are not effective replacements for steroids. Buchu and uva ursi may act as mild diuretics, and hops as a mild sedative.]
Hot Stuff $25.95 for 1 pound	Bodybuilding supplement powder whose many exotic ingredients include pyroglutamate, dibencozide, yohimbe, smilax, gamma oryzanol, transferulic acid, and muyrapuama	Combining Hot Stuff with a weight-training program will add muscle, increase strength, and reduce fat. [Smilax is an extract of sarsaparilla root that can cause diarrhea, dehydration, and an increase in heart rate. There is no evidence that dibencozide is a true ergogenic aid.]

Table 15-5 (cont). "Ergogenic Aids"

Product/Price	Description	Claims and Comments
The Power Pill $21.95 for 90 tablets	Extremely potent "anabolic" containing trace minerals, amino acids, herbs, cofactors, orchic [testicular] tissue, and digestive enzymes	"When combined with intense training you will experience tremendous growth and strength never before possible." "The gains made with the POWER PILL are permanent." Safest, fastest, and most effective way to achieve huge, hard muscularity and strength without harmful side effects ["Orchic" tissue, like all "glandulars," is rendered "impotent" by digestion.]
Green Magma USA $15.96 for 2.8 ounces, $24.00 for 300 tablets	Concentrated barley juice powder	Pure water and Green Magma are virtually all that is needed to replenish and maintain one's body every day.
xCELL Energy Wafers $9.95 for 10 servings	"Designed to perfection," this "energy food" provides active women with 100% of the daily requirements for nine important vitamins plus iron and calcium for only 130 calories.	"No other energy food comes close to xCELL's nutrient to calorie ratio because no other food is made like xCELL." [This claim is not just dubious, but trivial, since these nutrients can be obtained in comparable quantities at a negligible caloric "cost" in the form of one or two pills. For nutritional value, certain breakfast cereals are a much better buy.]
"Flower pollen" $18.00 for 100 tablets	Organic, living food used by bodybuilders and thousands of Europeans as a multivitamin	Used in animal breeding for stud power and increased sperm count; contains hundreds of nutrients, vitamins, amino acids, and enzymes. [What matters is not the number or variety of nutrients, but the amounts of essential ones. Enzyme content is irrelevant. Pollen has no significant therapeutic or nutritive value, and may cause allergic reactions.]

though," it states in boldface, "just solid steady gains as long as you also train hard and eat properly." Of course, the ad fails to mention that hard training and proper eating will do the job just as well without the product.

Often the name of a product implies a claim related to health or physical fitness. For example, the name of an herbal preparation—*Test R' Own 1000*—suggests the male hormone testosterone, an anabolic steroid. Another product is called *Ripped Fast* (see table). In *Exercise For Men Only*, a full-page ad for *Ripped Fast* begins: "No matter what they say, Looks Count! Your entire sexual identity may rest in how good you look to the opposite sex."

The "name game" is by no means a new trend. The first court trial under the Pure Food and Drugs Act of 1906, forerunner of today's Food, Drug, and Cosmetic Act, involved a product called *Cuforhedake Brane-Fude*.

A full-page ad in *Muscular Development*—for "The Most Explosive Muscle Building/Fat Loss System Ever!"—includes photos of two unidentified men. The photos are labeled weeks 1, 4, and 8. At first glance, the photos suggest impressive changes in physique. But closer analysis reveals: (1) both men look pale and have chest hair only in the "Week 1" photos, which are the brightest; (2) their "Week 1" and "Week 4" postures are different; and (3) their skin looks oily only in the "Week 8" photos. Further, the system includes a training program. Such a program and cosmetic adjustments are sufficient to account for the apparent changes in physique.

MuscleMag International is a monthly replete with ads for nutritional ergogenic aids. Ironically, it published a full-page ad that states:

> Did you know that as many as 8 out of 10 nutritional supplements don't contain what the manufacturers claim, much less do what their advertisers boast? In fact, some supplements don't contain any of the ingredients that are listed on their label! Many others contain only 10% of what they are supposed to.

A classified ad in Joe Weider's *Muscle & Fitness* for a training-aid booklet bids: "Don't waste your money on supplements that don't work. Work your muscles not your wallet." Some of the ads in *Muscle & Fitness* for Weider sports nutrition products include the statement: "As with all supplements, use of this product will not promote faster or greater muscular gains." I couldn't have put it better myself.

In noting the uselessness of nutritional ergogenic aids, let us not assume that they are harmless. A recent study by the Federation of American Societies for Experimental Biology revealed that little scientific literature exists on the use of individual amino acids for enhancing bodily functions and that they have not been demonstrated to be safe. Most

Americans consume at least as much protein as they need. Although bodybuilders and endurance athletes may need above-RDA amounts of protein for the repair of muscle fibers stressed during exercise, their high caloric requirements nearly ensure adequacy of protein intake without supplementation.

Another popular and problematic food constituent is boron, a supposed "supernutrient" promoted as an ergogenic aid, aphrodisiac, and arthritis remedy. Boron supplements have been marketed since the late 1980s. The mineral is available as a single-nutrient supplement and as an ingredient of products geared toward bodybuilders. However, in the May/June 1992 issue of *Nutrition Today*, pivotal boron researcher Forrest H. Nielsen, Ph.D., notes: (1) it seems fallacious to state that boron supplementation increases increases lean body mass and strength in humans; (2) a boron intake of 1 mg per day seems appropriate; (3) 10 mg of boron can be obtained daily through diet alone; and (4) toxic intakes of boron can easily occur through the excessive use of supplements. Foods high in boron include noncitrus fruits, leafy vegetables, nuts, and legumes.

Chromium is another mineral popular with fitness-seekers because of the claim that it is "anabolic." Unlike boron, chromium is an essential nutrient. Good food sources include apples, brown rice, chicken, chickpeas, cocoa, corn flakes, mushrooms, peanuts, raisins, spaghetti, and whole-wheat bread. Chromium is a component of a food constituent called glucose tolerance factor (GTF). Both GTF and chromium promote the interaction of insulin with cell surface receptors. This enables glucose to pass into the cells, where it is "burned" for energy. Exercise and the ingestion of simple sugars increase losses of chromium in the urine, hence the concern that athletes may be prone to a suboptimal chromium status. However, a recent review article in the *International Journal of Sports Medicine* concluded that adding chromium to the diet of normal healthy athletes is unlikely to produce significant muscle growth.

Government researchers who surveyed single issues of twelve popular health and bodybuilding magazines noted many ingredients they considered unusual or unidentifiable. No ingredients were listed for more than one fifth of the 311 products they counted, and for most listed ingredients, amounts were not indicated. Dosages were suggested in fewer than 25 percent of the instances wherein ingredients were listed. For most of the ingredients with suggested dosages, no RDA exists. One product contained a pharmacologic dose of folic acid—twenty-five times the U.S. RDA. High levels of folic acid can mask symptoms of pernicious anemia, a potentially fatal disease that can lead to irreversible nerve damage. The study was published in the August 26, 1992, *Journal of the American Medical Association,*

About a hundred companies market "ergogenic aids." In May 1992, the New York City Department of Consumer Affairs issued Notices of Violation to six of them. Manufacturers contacted by the department were unable to provide a single published report from a scientific journal to back the fitness-related claims they make for their products. The entire industry appears to be a scam.

"Anti-Aging" Products

Biogenetics Food Corporation, headquartered in Naples, Florida, sent me an information packet on *Bioguard* and *Bioguard Plus.* These are wheat-sprout supplements said to be "derived from special strains of wheat which are Biodynamically sprouted in a unique oxygen and nutrient-rich hydroponic environment." A flyer states: "Whole food antioxidant enzyme support from Biogenetics concentrated sprout products offers a powerful tool in the prevention and management of a broad range of free radical-induced tissue damage." In one brochure, the supposed utility of both products appears to rest largely in their proportion of antioxidant enzymes such as superoxide dismutase (SOD). Enzymes are proteins and are digested as such; they are absorbed in the form of constituent amino acids and small peptides, thus losing whatever antioxidant properties they might have possessed before being dismembered. However, the mailings I received emphasized nutritional "support" of antioxidant enzymes, rather than antioxidant enzyme *content.*

The initial information packet included a booklet titled "Antioxidant Enzyme Nutritional Support," by Zane Baranowski, CN, BCNC. The booklet cites the "obvious" limitations of "isolated" antioxidant enzyme supplements, including "poor stability" and "difficult absorbability." Instead, the author plays up the antioxidant content of sprouts. He concludes: "Whole food antioxidant enzyme support is the perfect adjunct to any nutritional protocol focused upon prevention, detoxification, environmental protection, longevity, and composure in the face of adversity."

Curious about the initials following his name, I called Biogenetics via its toll-free number and was advised to call the author directly via another toll-free number. Zane answered the phone, and our conversation lasted for about two hours. The initials after his name, he explained, stand for "Certified Nutritionist" and "Board Certified Nutrition Consultant." The

Table 13-6. "Anti-Aging" Products

Product/Price	Description	Claims and Comments
Bioguard About $26 for 1-month supply Bioguard Plus About $29.00 for 1- month supply	Wheat-sprout tablets and caplets. Bioguard is grown to emphasize superoxide dismutase and catalase, Bioguard Plus to emphasize a broader spectrum of antioxidant enzymes.	Unique whole food complexes containing natural bioactive precursors favorable for antioxidant enzyme requirements ("Whole Food Solutions to Free Radical Pollution")
Cervital $17.20 for 100 tablets, $37 for 250 tablets	Exclusive European antioxidant product containing vitamins A, B-6, C, and E; selenium; zinc; and pollen extract	Helps slow down the visible and not-so-visible signs of aging by fighting harmful free radicals
Pyc-C About $25.00 for 60 capsules	25 mg pycnogenol, 500 mg corn-free vitamin C, 25 mg calcium, 25 mg magnesium, and 1 mg zinc. "Pycnogenol" is the trade name for a bioflavonoid-containing concentrate of substances found in grape seeds and maritime pine bark.	Beautifies skin, slows aging, and fortifies vessels. Pycnogenol is largely composed of natural antioxidants nearly twenty times more effective than vitamin C in vitro at trapping free radicals.
Cell Guard $26.50 for 60 tablets	Potentiator complex containing coenzyme Q10, methionine, 9 vitamins, 3 minerals 4 adaptogenic herbs, and dimethylglycine (DMG)	Neutralizes free radicals that damage the body's immunity; helps the body's vitality
Living Waters $13.50 for 4 ounces	Water electromagnetically imprinted with a 28-organism yogurt microculture used by the long-lived people of Soviet Georgia for thousands of years	[No specific claims made. Probably a homeopathic placebo.]
Bogdana Rejuvenating Formula $55.00 for 5 ounces $26.00 for 1-month supply	Liquid high-energy supplement based on quantum physics. Contains 150 vitamins, minerals, amino acids, and proteins, plus pure energy. Primary ingredients are honey, blackstrap molasses, predigested yeast, and collagen [a low-quality protein familiar as gelatin].	Cleanses toxins out of the body; immunity booster; ergogenic aid; takes into account the nutritional needs of the body's magnetic fields; promotes balance in life. A magnetic resonance is incorporated to help the body find appropriate targets.

"CN" credential was awarded to him, he said, by the National Institute of Nutritional Education (NINE), and the "BCNC" had come from the American Board of Nutritional and Naturopathic Certification, but was "not current." He had earned them by passing exams, he said, but he readily admitted that neither organization was accredited or "recognized." He suggested that the BCNC certificate amounted to a "nice thing on my wall," and used an expletive to indicate its meaning. Otherwise, he had finished one year of college without a major. Of *Bioguard* he said: "Our product doesn't have any SOD in it, and if it did, who knows if it's absorbable?"

The free-radical theory of aging is but one of many theories concerning the aging process. Free radicals are atoms or molecules with at least one unpaired electron. Unpaired electrons render molecules such as ozone highly reactive and, thus, destructive. Free radicals derive both from the environment and from metabolism. The free-radical theory holds that aging occurs with gradually increasing accumulation of micro-injuries induced by free radicals. Antioxidant supplements and drugs are promoted as free-radical quenchers or "scavengers." Supplementation advocates claim that ingestion of antioxidant vitamins and minerals can retard aging through the interruption of free-radical chain reactions. But no vitamin or drug has been proven to significantly extend the maximum life span of any mammal, including humans.

It may be significant that researchers who studied vitamin consumption by readers of *Prevention* magazine over age sixty-five found no dose-response relationship between mortality and supplementation levels. In this study, increased mortality was observed in people who had consumed very high levels of vitamin E—more than 1,000 IU per day. Although this may reflect an attraction for less healthy persons to large doses of vitamins, it may also reflect some long-range vitamin toxicity.

The January 1992 *Consumer Reports* quotes Professor Caleb Finch of the University of Southern California: "Peculiar things happen when you dump chemicals in your body. Each has its own effect, and there's no way to predict the interactions or the long-term consequences."

How to Spot a Rip-off

An item in a 1992 issue of another consumer-protection publication cites a mail-order ad for a "solid-state compact food server" costing $39.95, which turned out to be a spoon. In this case the fraud is obvious. With pills, potions, and powders, the fraud may not be obvious because it is difficult to measure the impact of a "nutritional" product without double-blind studies. The only practical way for an individual to determine whether a health product can work as advertised is to examine the claims in light of established scientific evidence. The following questions may provoke healthy consumer skepticism:

- *Does the ad provide any explicit, practical information?* Poetic ads are often a tip-off that the product is a placebo or a grossly overpriced source of nutrients. It might be useful to know the names of the major ingredients, the recommended dose, the amount of each major ingredient per dose, whether the product is expiration-dated, and the company's refund policy. Are any of the ingredients exotic? Are the exotic ingredients described in any legitimate reference book on medicine, nutrition, foods, food technology, or herbs?

- *Is the company reputable?* One might well wonder about the presence of contaminants and about the actual amounts, potency, safety, bioavailability, and very presence of the listed ingredients.

- *Do any of the ingredients have known side effects?* Are there contra-indications for any of them? Is the product a food item, a nutritional supplement, a drug, or a placebo? Even some water-soluble vitamins have known side effects, and a nontraditional food item previously absent from one's diet may prove allergenic or otherwise disagree-able.

- *Are the claims made for the product plausible on the basis of its ingredients?* Have the claims been tested scientifically? If so, are they supported or negated by the evidence, or are the findings equivocal? If you cannot answer these questions confidently, skip the product.

- *Are your reasonable expectations adequate grounds for buying the product at the advertised price?* Are the ingredients available in a less expensive, more effective, or more palatable form? For example, a basket of fresh fruit is likely to be less expensive, more nutritious, tastier, and safer than a bottle of the "potassium mineral supplement" *Km.*

In the May 1992 issue of his science newsletter, *Probe,* investigative reporter David Zimmerman opines that millions of Americans are need-lessly ingesting vitamin supplements in part because of

personal insecurity, boosted by economic hard times and social demoralization. We sense that many people are looking for meth-ods that are close in—close to the chest—that they can use, and control, to safeguard and better their lives. So, swallowing extra large amounts of these vital chemicals has the same urgency—and may confer the same sense of security—as eating sacramental food.

In 1991, the American Council on Science and Health published "Quackery By Mail," a report written by consumer health advocate Stephen Barrett, M.D. Dr. Barrett estimates that Americans spend between 50 and 150 million dollars a year on mail-order "health" products. He warns:

- Be very skeptical of advertising claims for mail-order "health" products. Almost all such products are misrepresented.

- Don't be misled by the promise of a "money-back guarantee." There is no reason to believe that the guarantee is any better than the product.

- No product can "melt away fat" or cause effortless weight loss.

- No mail-order product can erase scars, wrinkles, or "cellulite."

- No device can selectively reduce one part of your body.

- No mail-order product can increase bust or penis size.

- No mail-order product can prevent or cure hair loss.

- No mail-order nutrient product can increase stamina or endurance or increase strength or muscle mass.

- No nutrient product can "prevent aging" or prolong life.

- No nutrient product can prevent senility or increase memory.

- No pill can increase sexual stimulation or pleasure.

- Musical tapes with "subliminal" messages can't do anything more for physical or mental well-being than listening to ordinary music.

- In fact, so few mail-order health products work as advertised that you should never buy one without medical advice.

The Bottom Line

It appears that most if not all nutrition-related "health" products sold through periodical ads are: (1) safe but useless, (2) dangerous over the long term, or (3) at best, luxuries of questionable utility. Buying nutrition-related products by mail is both risky and unnecessary.

14

Chiropractic Nutrition: The "Supplement Underground"

The "Pushers"

As reported in the July 1989 *Journal of the American Dietetic Association*, several registered dietitians and a chiropractor mailed a questionnaire to the entire membership of the San Francisco Bay Area Chiropractic Society. They found that nearly all of the one hundred respondents counseled their patients on nutrition, and that most did so routinely. They also found that more of these chiropractors were familiar with naturopathic education than with the educational backgrounds of registered dietitians. In the same year, a spokesperson for Douglas Laboratories, which sells nutritional products only to chiropractors, stated that "roughly 65% of all chiropractors are dispensing nutritional products, and more of them are doing it every day."

Chiropractic is based upon the belief that most ailments are the result of spinal problems. The "discovery" of chiropractic is attributed to Daniel David Palmer, a grocer and "magnetic healer" who practiced in Davenport, Iowa. Palmer believed that a vital force—which he termed the "Innate"—expressed itself through the nervous system. In 1895 he concluded that he had restored the hearing of a partially deaf janitor by "adjusting" a bump on his spine. Not long afterward he decided that the basic cause of disease is "nerve interference" caused by misaligned spinal bones, which could be adjusted back into place by hand.

In *Alternative Medicine and Religious Life (1989)*, philosophy professor Robert C. Fuller notes:

213

Daniel associated with a good many spiritualists from whom he picked up a number of metaphysical terms and metaphors for humanity's participation in a higher order of things. Even well into his chiropractic days he simply took for granted that "we are surrounded with an aura" and . . . are intimately connected with nonmaterial forces.

Today's 45,000+ chiropractors can be divided into two broad philosophical camps: "straights" and "mixers." Straights tend to cling to Palmer's basic doctrine that most disease is caused by misaligned vertebrae ("subluxations") and thus can be cured by "adjusting" the spine. Mixers acknowledge that germs, hormones, and other factors play a role in disease, but they tend to regard mechanical disturbances of the nervous system as the underlying cause. In addition to spinal manipulation, mixers may use nutritional methods and various forms of physiotherapy (heat, cold, traction, exercise, massage, and ultrasound).

Although some scientific nutrition concepts are taught in chiropractic schools, many ideas that chiropractors absorb—in school and afterwards— are as unscientific as their basic theory of disease. Chiropractors who give nutritional advice typically recommend dietary supplements that are unnecessary or are inappropriate for treatment of the patient's health problem. Much of the advice they give is acquired at seminars given by companies that market "nutritional products" exclusively or primarily to chiropractors. Speakers at the seminars typically make claims for the products that would not be legal on product labels because they are false or unproven. (It is a federal crime for a manufacturer to claim that a product can prevent, cure, mitigate, or treat a health problem unless the product is regarded by experts as safe and effective for that purpose.) Thus the seminars serve as a conduit for illegal claims hidden from government regulators.

Murray the "Mixer"

One of chiropractic's most active proponents of supplement-prescribing is retired chiropractor Richard R. Murray. A seminar flyer exalts him as "the dean of contemporary clinical nutrition," an "internationally acclaimed researcher, teacher, and consultant," and a life-long friend and colleague of Dr. Royal Lee.

Royal S. Lee was a nonpracticing dentist who co-founded the National Health Federation (a "health food" industry advocacy group), started a food supplement company, and organized the Lee Foundation for Nutritional Research, a prolific distributor of health and nutrition literature. One of Lee's principles was: "A fact need not be 'proved' to be useful." In 1962, Lee and the vitamin company he ran were found guilty of misbranding 115 special dietary products by making false claims for the treatment of more than five hundred diseases and conditions. Lee received a one-year suspended prison term and was fined $7,000. In 1963, a prominent FDA official said Lee was "probably the largest publisher of unreliable and false nutritional information in the world." Lee died in 1967, but the company is still marketing many of the same products—mainly through chiropractors.

Supplements said to be researched and formulated by Murray are now marketed by Nutri-West, a company headquartered in Douglas, Wyoming. Nutri-West promotes applied kinesiology and sponsors seminars given by Murray across the United States. Berman Chiropractic Supply (BCS) in Florida, New York, is one of thirteen Nutri-West distributors in the United States, Canada, and England. BCS markets Murray's formulations and similar products to chiropractors and other practitioners in nine northeastern states.

In 1987, a prominent consumer reporter attended a BCS-sponsored seminar and received a large book listing 142 conditions ranging from acidosis to whooping cough and recommending Nutri-West supplements for each one. The speaker described a scheme for billing insurance companies for dubious laboratory tests.

During the same year, BCS distributed copies of Nutri-West's ten-page "Professional Order Form" to members of the American Nutrimedical Association, many of whose members sport dubious credentials and engage in unscientific nutrition practices (see Chapter 12). The order form listed more than two hundred "glandular," enzyme, and herbal products, dietary supplements, "specialty items," and "core level products." Although the literature doesn't specify how the products should be used, many were named after organs of the body (e.g., *Cardio-Lymph Chelate, Adreno-Lymph*, and *Core Level Heart*).

In 1991, I received a schedule of BCS-sponsored seminars to be given by Murray that year. The mailing also included a BCS information sheet for "health care professionals," which associated ten of his formulations with medical problems: gout (*ARTHRO-G*), osteoarthritis (*ARTHRO-O*), rheumatoid arthritis (*ARTHRO-R*), multiple sclerosis (*BIOLAC*), diabetes and hypoglycemia (*CARBO-MET*), Alzheimer's disease (*NEURO TONE*), female sexual dysfunction (*FEM VITEX*), impotence (*HERBAL*

VITEX), and anxiety (*STRESS PAN F* for females, *STRESS PAN M* for males). *FEM DEL* is associated with "young female breast development."

I registered for a seminar, but was notified that it had been canceled because Murray had had a serious accident followed by the amputation of his right leg. The letter was signed by Judith A. DeCava, C.N.C. (The initials after her name stand for "Certified Nutrition Consultant," a "credential" without scientific, professional, or academic significance.) Murray, she wrote, "has been recuperating at an excellent rate; his doctors don't understand it! Naturally, the nutritional support he has been using has been of tremendous assistance."

A One-Ring Biochemical Circus

My opportunity to attend a Murray seminar finally came in mid-1992, when a ten-hour "Masters Series" seminar was held in a basement room at the LaGuardia Marriott Hotel in New York City on June 27 and 28. The pre-registration cost for doctors was $175. About fifty people attended. In the back of the room, supplements and product literature were available for sale, with a limited amount of literature offered without charge. I selected a flyer, a magazine, and a Nutri-West/Micro-West catalog.

The flyer described seventeen products formulated by Murray, and nearly four dozen additional homeopathic and nutritional products "for the yuks"—"the answer to all of your patient's blahs."

The magazine was the January/February issue of *The Journal of the National Academy of Research Biochemists*. Its twenty-eight pages contained three major articles, two of which were written by Murray. Its cover states that the academy is "Dedicated to the Preservation and Advancement of Truth in the Field of Nutrition." Its masthead states that the academy is owned by the James Homer Russell Foundation and that unlicensed individuals who use the information in the journal for diagnosing or treating any symptom or ailment could be violating civil or criminal laws. One of the journal's ads is for a book called *How to Practice Nutritional Counseling Without Being Guilty Of Practicing Medicine Without A License.*

The Micro-West catalog lists and describes indications for seventy-five liquid homeopathic "drugs," including ear drops, hand lotion, mouthwash, and "remedies" for everything from "diabetes involvement" to "free radical toxicity." Each one-ounce bottle costs doctors $6; the suggested retail price is $12—a 100 percent markup.

Each attendee was given a four-page patient handout prepared by R. Murray and Associates, Inc., and a loose-leaf binder labeled "Berman Chiropractic Supply." The former included an "adjunctive nutritional schedule" worksheet designed to facilitate the "suggesting" and pricing of supplementation regimens. But the first page of the handout included the disclaimer:

Be advised that the suggested nutritional program . . . is not intended as primary therapy for any disease or symptom but is an adjunctive schedule of nutrients (food concentrates) provided solely to upgrade the quality of foods in the diet in order to supply good nutrition for supporting the physiological and biochemical processes of the human body.

The handout's "General Dietary Suggestions" encourage consumption of sea salt, raw milk from cows or goats, raw nuts and seeds, nonhydrogenated peanut butter, and a variety of "health foods." They call for avoidance of artificial sweeteners, pasteurized milk, other common foods, and "high potency vitamins which are mostly fractions of vitamin complexes or synthetic." The loose-leaf binder contained a Nutri-West catalog, ten commentaries by Murray on subjects ranging from nutritional treatment of osteoarthritis to "subclinical" beriberi, and ten related product descriptions ("adjunctive tips") by Judith DeCava, C.N.C. Most of the commentaries and descriptions are marked "For Clinicians Only" or "For Physicians Only."

The seminar was a one-man show with an emphasis on biochemistry—of a sort. Murray's teaching style involved much verbatim quoting of articles he had on hand, references to his commentaries, use of a markerboard, and tongue-in-cheek humor. He is a smooth talker who impressed me as being a very well-read businessman. During the registration period, he made his negative position clear on vaccinations and fluoridation. With regard to hepatitis, he pronounced: "The test isn't worth a nickel, and the vaccine is worse. Somebody wants to kill us all." An attendee added: "For money." Another said: "They want to do it slow, though, so they can extract every penny out of you." Then Murray cited a Dutch doctor's book, which, he said, shows that "there's definite information that fluoride is a mind-control drug that causes people who drink fluoridated water to be docile and [not really] care if they're controlled by other people." According to Murray, the book also shows that mind control has been "one of the basic underlying purposes of water fluoridation" since its inception.

BCS president Jerry Berman formally introduced Murray, who thereupon recounted the events that had led to the loss of his right leg.

Murray said he had quit practicing chiropractic in 1984. However, a woman with cerebral palsy talked him into treating her. Much to Murray's surprise, her symptoms were "reduced" after just five days of "inpatient" chiropractic and nutritional treatment he had administered in his house. The woman subsequently referred other persons with cerebral palsy to him, and Murray "could not believe" the resulting changes in them. So he began building an office near St. Louis, Missouri, to accommodate residential treatment of cerebral palsy patients.

One December night he was scrubbing tiles in the new office. Wearing heavy socks, he went outside without shoes to get something from his car. As he opened the car door, he accidentally stepped on a pile of lumber and twisted his ankle, which he bandaged upon his return to the office. After about twelve days of limping around with what he thought was a sprained ankle, Murray decided it wasn't healing, probably because he had been on his feet too much. So he soaked his ankle in Epsom salts and water and then discovered a splinter of wood embedded in the crumpled flesh of his heel. He removed it and figured he'd soon be okay, but his condition worsened until he became delirious and disoriented. When his wife phoned him at the office, she became concerned and contacted one of his employees, who "conned" Murray into going to the hospital. A diagnosis of gangrene led to the amputation of his leg the following morning.

Murray rationalized:

> Nevertheless, I think it saved my life, 'cause as I mentioned earlier, I'd been running as fast as I could go for fifty years. I was worn-out, I couldn't hardly do a six-hour seminar without being totally exhausted, and everything was completely trying. [Now] I can give ten- or twelve-hour seminars again and still feel good. So the four-month rest at Veterans Hospital, I think, saved my life. So I lost my leg, but I saved my life.

An attendee inquired whether the splinter had come from chemically treated lumber. Murray said he didn't know, but added that his surgeon had raised that suspicion.

"The Secret of Life"

Murray gave us his private telephone number and invited us to call him for consultations at a cost of $25 per "nutritional schedule." He said of the fee: "If the patient dies, we won't talk about it." Murray explained the instructions that had been on the marker-board since my arrival:

If I had a patient come into my office and they said: "Dr. Murray, I have nothing wrong with me. I'm in perfect health. What should I do to maintain status quo?" ... I would put them on this schedule:

Upon Arising	*Before 2 Meals*	*After Eve Meal*
4 Calac	1 Biostress-B	1 Wht. Grm. Oil 770
1 Biolac	1 Carbomet	
	1 Minbal	

Listed on the marker-board were six supplements, the first five of which are tablets formulated by Murray: *CALAC*, containing calcium lactate and magnesium; *BIOLAC*, containing 190 mg of lactose "derived from a natural source"; *BIOSTRESS-B*, containing thiamine, primary yeast, rice bran, and wheat germ; *CARBO-MET*, containing bovine gland concentrates, minerals, and herbs; *MINBAL*, containing calcium lactate, magnesium, and alfalfa; and capsules containing 770 mg of wheat germ oil. The total monthly cost of this basic, "preventative" regimen is about $36.

"Now in order to make sure that you profit from this seminar," Murray said later, "I'm going to tell you the secret of life." He thereupon referred us to one of his commentaries in the loose-leaf binder, titled "Vitex, Vitality Complex." "This," he declared, "is a formula for male impotency." He further stated:

I said I was gonna make your visit here profitable. You could go home with nothing but two dozen of these, and you can build your practice. Once your male patient, over thirty-five, takes *Herbal Vitex*, he will never quit. I have an 82-year-old patient in St. Louis, and I told him he didn't need three a day, and he said: "I'll take three a day for the rest of my life." And I said: "Well, you're not gonna live too long, so it won't matter; you're not gonna spend that much money." But, nevertheless, I can't get anyone off of it once I put them on it.

According to the commentary, *Herbal Vitex* is composed of yohimbe bark, damiana, gotu kola, hawthorne berries, beet root, and Korean ginseng. Murray directed our attention to two paragraphs in the commentary citing a favorable report published in *The Lancet* on yohimbine—a constituent of yohimbe. After he recited the alleged benefits of taking yohimbine, an anti-amalgamist dentist seated to my left asked him if *Herbal Vitex* contained it. Murray replied that it contained yohimbe bark, not the extract yohimbine, which is a prescription drug. But he added: "They find that the whole works better than the part." He left unmentioned the possible side effects of yohimbe tea listed in the commentary:

"lethargic debility of the limbs, restlessness, chills, some nausea and vertigo." Murray told us that the product has been endorsed by Jim Bakker, Jimmy Swaggart, Mike Tyson, Pee-wee Herman, and Jessica Hahn. (All five have been involved in sex scandals, but Murray did not specify any connection with taking the product.) When should one stop taking the product? Murray said he tells doctors who ask him this question to quit when they're jailed on a charge of rape.

"Vitamin B-complex deficiency syndrome," he said, exists in about 33 to 50 percent of patients. "Unusual weakness and fatigue is the first symptom of B-complex deficiency." He stated that every patient should take at least two *Biostress-B* tablets per day.

Murray termed the diet/serum cholesterol/heart disease connection a "scam"—"nonsense" that started with the Framingham Heart Study. "A high cholesterol," he declared, "means over 330." He said that it's been well known for fifty years that "a patient over forty years of age would normally have a normal serum cholesterol of 240 to 330." (Of course, the relevant question is not "What level is normal?" but "What level is healthful?" The National Cholesterol Education Program classifies serum total cholesterol levels below 200 mg/dl as desirable and levels 240 and above as high. Most persons with a level above 240 would be at high risk for developing coronary heart disease. A chiropractor who routinely assured patients not to worry about a cholesterol level between 240 and 330 would certainly be committing malpractice.)

A Procession of Fallacies

Murray indicated that one reason to use *CALAC* as he recommended is to boost immunity. He suggested that ionizable calcium be administered if a child has a fever. "How much ionized calcium is in the phagocyte," he claimed, "gives it its ability to do its job—that's the common denominator of phagocytosis capability." The second reason he gave for using *CALAC* is a supposed lack of convenient natural sources of ionizable calcium. Calcium chloride, he explained, is absent from tap water, and raw milk is very difficult to obtain. Pasteurization, he (incorrectly) claimed, renders the calcium in milk unabsorbable. Moreover, he intimated that the form of calcium in pasteurized milk could contribute to a calcium deficiency. He further claimed that persons not drinking raw milk or "good, deep well water uncontaminated by man" do not get enough calcium in their diet.

However, in addition to raw cow or goat milk, the dietary suggestions in his patient handout recommend cheeses that are "not processed," including "real" cottage cheese. Murray related the advice he had given to a pregnant patient and her husband during a "house call": "Anything that God made and man hasn't messed with is good to eat."

This advice is not only fallacious but potentially harmful. Calcium from milk is readily absorbed, and many water supplies contain significant amounts. Raw milk is a source of dangerous infection, and its sale is prohibited in many states and in interstate commerce.

The Epitome of Biochemical Ignorance?

Next, Murray talked about food enzymes and read a statement from one of his commentaries:

BIOCHEMICAL FACT: Enzymes are essential to food quality. Live foods—foods with their naturally-occurring enzymes intact are essential to life and health. Foods devoid of enzymes are dead foods which cannot sustain life and health. For anyone to say otherwise is the epitome of biochemical ignorance.

At the risk of "epitomizing" biochemical ignorance, I would like to supply a few facts. First, some enzymes affect food quality adversely. For example, in the presence of air or oxygen, certain oxidases turn fruits and vegetables brown. Second, although enzymes are proteins, food enzymes are a negligible source of protein and are nutritionally insignificant. Third, while digestive enzymes can be medically useful, food enzymes have no such utility when consumed as part of food. Like all other proteins, they are absorbed in the form of their constituent amino acids and small peptides, thus losing whatever properties they might have possessed before being dismembered. Even if they could be absorbed intact, enzymes from plants would have little or no effect on human biochemistry.

Murray, of course, differs with this view. "Enzymes are the key, and live vitamins with enzymes intact and minerals are essential to proper nutrition," he told us. "When you pasteurize milk, you destroy forty-seven enzymes." He added that the lactose in raw milk is necessary for bone formation, but that pasteurization renders it unusable by changing its molecular configuration. He further stated that galactose (a constituent of lactose) is essential for the maintenance and repair of the myelin sheath. He had had great results with multiple sclerosis patients in Florida, he said, until the state had made raw milk unavailable. "The dirtiest raw milk," he averred, "is probably cleaner than the cleanest pasteurized." However, he cited one "disadvantage": "When you drink raw milk, you don't attain enough growth to become a professional basketball player." Murray summarized his position: "As the age of devitalized food has progressed, our men are getting taller and taller, and weaker and weaker." He recommended that pasteurized milk be excluded from the diets of multiple sclerosis patients, and that they be given *BIOLAC*. (The amount of lactose in a pint of milk is equivalent to one hundred *BIOLAC* tablets.)

Some *Don't* Like It Hot

"People are allergic to anything and everything that's poison," Murray declared, "and just about everything we eat today is poison: everything we eat is contaminated with poisons." He urged us not to use microwave ovens and to discourage our patients from using them. He further stated:

> What does your microwave do? It destroys all the enzyme activity that might be left in your food. If there was any left at all, it's gone after you microwave. And I used to tell people that . . . the only problem with microwave is you were destroying any life that was left in [the food]. . . . So, if you got a microwave oven, sell it to your neighbor that you don't like.

"Cooked food disease is one of our major plagues," he asserted. "Distilled water is a thousand times better than tap water, but distilled water, when it's heated above 194 degrees Fahrenheit, becomes toxic to the human biochemistry." Boiled water, he said, causes "physiological leukocytosis, indicating that the heated water is toxic." "You should start your meal with raw foods, because," he claimed, "there are enzymes in raw food that have the effect of detoxifying cooked foods—to some degree. . . . So it's a good idea to have raw foods previous to cooked foods."

I asked Murray whether any mechanism had been proposed to explain the (alleged) toxicity of distilled water. He replied simply that natural substances subjected to heat become toxic and trigger leukocytosis. "So pure H_2O is toxic?" I pressed—whereupon the attendee across the aisle from me broke in: "There's no such thing as pure H_2O except in the laboratory. Water is never pure. When you distill it, you change the polarity, you change the electromagnetic field, you make it a vacuum." Murray agreed, adding: "You have different isomers that the body can't handle."

The Bottom Line

Very few chiropractors are bona fide experts in scientific nutrition. No nutrition courses are required during pre-chiropractic study, and the scope and quality of nutrition courses differ from from one chiropractic college to another. While the American Chiropractic Board of Nutrition offers a program leading to "certification" in nutrition, this process does not turn chiropractors into experts.

Richard R. Murray is certainly not a nutrition expert. Sounding like biochemical spiritism, his teachings range from the unproven and false to those that the scientific nutritionists would find ludicrous. BCS and similar companies are using seminars like Murray's to promote dubious products and to transmit unproven claims that would not be legal on product labels.

Do you think that chiropractors who embrace teachings such as Murray's are likely to provide patients with a rational form of health care?

15

"Nontraditional" Health Education: Reading, Writing, and Religion

Health Education or Cultism?

"Alternative" medicine advocates appear at least as interested in the quality of an imagined "vital principle" in food as they are in the effects of actual food constituents. I seriously doubt that self-styled "nutritional herbalists" or "herbal nutritionists" and kindred counterculturists and pseudoprofessionals are able to recognize the often subtle, slowly worsening side effects of their "supplements." Yet, the eleventh edition of *Bear's Guide to Earning College Degrees Non-Traditionally* (1992) describes twenty-five unaccredited "health-related" schools in one chapter alone; other dubious health-related educational programs are described in three other chapters. Moreover, these represent just a fraction of the myriad enterprises offering dubious healthcare-related degrees, diplomas, certificates, and titles to virtually anyone willing to pay.

A cult may be defined as an unscientific system that encourages obsessive devotion to a person or an ideal. It appears that most of these nontraditional schools foster cultism. The table on the next page outlines several nutrition-related cults.

Almost an Herbalist

Educational opportunities abound for religionists and assorted paranormalists seeking (ostensibly) secular occupations compatible with (and

225

Unscientific Nutrition Systems
Each of these systems fits the definition of a cult.

System	Basis for Diet	Primary Food	Religious Roots	Designation for "Vital Principle"
Anthro-posophy	Teachings of "clairvoyant" Rudolf Steiner	All foods of the plant kingdom, "biodynamically grown"	Christianity Rosicrucianism Theosophy	No single equivalent, but refers to "soul" and "spirit"
Ayurveda	So-called constitutional types	Grains, ghee (clarified butter), and specific vegetables, all preferably heated or cooked. Maharishi Amrit Kalash is advertised as "the perfect nutritional food."	Hinduism	Prana
Edgar Cayce tradition	Cayce's "psychic readings"	All foods of the plant kingdom	Christianity Theosophy	Soul
Gerson therapy	Empiricism	Fresh "juices" composed of "organically grown" fruits and vegetables		Soul
Km/Pathway Nutrition System	Empiricism	Km	Theism	None
Macrobiotics	George Ohsawa's version of traditional Chinese cosmology	Brown rice	Zen Buddhism Hinduism Shinto	Ch'i (ki)
Natural Hygiene	Herbert Shelton's food categorizations	Raw vegetables, raw fruits, and raw nuts	Presbyterianism	Essence, life force
Nutripathy	So-called "proper food combining" (à la Shelton) and "metabolism types"	"Natural," "live," and "organically grown" foods	Christianity	Life force

apt to strengthen) their beliefs. Herbs may be broadly defined as plants believed to have culinary or therapeutic utility. In the field of nutrition and dietetics, herbs are properly used only as flavoring agents or garnishes, or for preparing liquid refreshment, such as an herbal tea. In the health marketplace, however, many herbs are promoted and used as remedies.

Emerson College of Herbology Ltd. in Ontario, Canada, established in 1975, is described in *Bear's Guide* in the chapter on "Medical and Health-Related Schools." In November 1989, I sent Emerson a check for $225—the prepayment fee for a correspondence course in "Scientific Herbology" consisting of thirty-three lessons composed by Prof. J.E. (Jack) Thuna, M.H., D.C., N.D. Today the cost is at least $325. Emerson's prospectus states:

> Take as much time as necessary to complete your Course, however the sooner you finish, the quicker you will be able to profit.
>
> On completion of the Course and having satisfactorily passed the questions in each lesson and the final examination with a "grading" percentage of 75%, you will be awarded a handsome DIPLOMA designating you as a qualified MASTER OF HERBOLOGY [M.H.].
>
> Those receiving a grading percentage of 85% or more throughout the course, will be eligible for admittance to the Research Council on Botanic Medicine as a Research Member (without extra cost). You will receive an official Certificate of Membership for framing.

Emerson's motto is: "Health is wealth. Herbs give health." The meandering lessons are marked by bombast, invective, and hyperbole. The statements below are excerpted from just the first nine lessons.

• This course of study is not like anything that has gone before.

• This lecture is only introductory serving to foreshadow the joy and delight you will experience in the course which we believe will pilot you quickly to honor and greatness, to say nothing of financial success.

• Nature is ever young and beautiful, ever vibrant with life and more life—why not man?

• During this course some of your more or less deep-seated convictions and beliefs are going to receive some severe jolts.

• We have not finished with oxygen and we never shall finish with it, because *oxygen* is the very *BREATH of LIFE*.

• The medical doctors are so totally ignorant of Nature's remedies that not one of them could stand before you in a court of law after you have acquired the knowledge of Herb Therapy embodied in this course. Your answers to their questions or plaints would make any one of them appear to be so ignorant before the Judge or Jury that you could not lose your case, and if you won, you would be famous overnight and could easily obtain an injunction against them which would make you free to practice Herbalism in any of the United States.

The lesson books are accompanied by short-answer quizzes. The quiz questions include: (1) What are the three "LIFE giving" potassium compounds and why are they so important? (2) For what conditions would you recommend the infusion of geranium root? (3) What are the virtues of black walnut leaves? (4) How would you prepare the salve of marigold? (5) What does all earth life depend on? (6) How would you recommend the blackberry plant for internal and external uses in the treatment of gout and arthritis? (7) Why is it so vital that you know the chemical constituents of herbs?

I experienced neither the joy nor the delight promised in the first tedious lesson, and so, less than a quarter of the way through the course, I requested a partial refund. My request was denied.

Some herbalists simply cultivate or collect herbs and make no claim to expertise in health care. Those who purport to specialize in the medicinal or "healing" uses of herbs may call themselves herbalists, herbologists, medical herbalists, or herb doctors. Most such practitioners have no training whatsoever either in scientific diagnosis or in pharmacognosy, a respectable branch of pharmacology focused on drugs in their crude or natural state. Rather, their "knowledge" is rooted in folklore, anecdotes, theism, and such vitalistic concepts as homeopathy and the "Doctrine of Signatures." The latter holds that herbs and other living things have a unique quality or "vibration" revealed in their shape and/or color. Some ginseng roots, for example, resemble a human body with a phallus and thus are prized as agents of virility—a ridiculous notion. But then, herbalism is suffused with pseudosophisticated silliness. Forms of herbalism are taught in schools of "oriental medicine" and naturopathy, and may be part of unscientific programs in massage therapy and nutrition.

Gary Null's Alma Mater

One of the speakers scheduled for the symposium held in October 1991 by the Foundation for the Advancement of Innovative Medicine (FAIM)) was

Gary Null (1945–), a popular "natural foods" advocate and author. (See Chapter 7 for information about FAIM.) The symposium flyer described him as a consumer advocate, an investigative reporter, and founder and director of the Health and Nutrition Certificate Program at Pratt Institute and the School of Visual Arts. He is in fact one of America's foremost promoters of dubious information about health and nutrition. During the 1980s, when I was a nutrition major at Pratt Institute, Null taught some courses there, but not in the department of nutrition and dietetics. In July 1992, Pratt's School of Professional Studies informed me that his program had been discontinued. Regrettably, I did not stay for Null's lecture at the FAIM symposium. I did, however, investigate the source of his doctorate.

The FAIM flyer states that Null holds a Ph.D. degree in human nutrition and public health sciences from Union Graduate School. The name of the school rang a bell, so I looked it up in *Bear's Guide.* "Union Graduate School" is the former name of The Union Institute in Cincinnati, Ohio, which adopted its current name in 1990. The school's literature says it was founded by ten college presidents in 1964 "as a vehicle for educational research and experimentation." Originally the Union for Experimenting Colleges and Universities, the institute is an accredited, nonprofit institution geared toward the "adult learner." It offers B.A., B.S., and Ph.D. degrees through individualized, short-residency programs in multifarious fields. Graduate tuition (1992–93) is $2,484 per quarter; board and lodgings (required at colloquia) impose additional expenses. A doctoral degree can be earned in two years. However, in *College Degrees by Mail* (1992), John Bear, Ph.D., writes that completion of the doctoral program usually takes about four years and can easily cost over $25,000.

The Union Institute's chief selling points are program flexibility and an interdisciplinary program. Its literature states: "By working in more than one field, learners have the opportunity to locate their ideas in a variety of frames of reference and thereby to participate in the emergence of new and vital constructs." Two goals of the doctoral program are personal development and social relevance. The school encourages students to "be keenly and continuously aware of the impact of the learning process on their lives" and defines doctoral study as "a force for social change."

Graduate school "learners" must design their own programs, develop them in consultation with faculty advisors, implement them, establish and chair their own doctoral committees, and prepare their own transcripts. There are no required courses, and faculty members function primarily as "facilitators." Only thirty-five days of residency are required: ten at an entry colloquium, fifteen at school-sponsored seminars, and ten "peer days." Peer days are interdisciplinary sessions arranged and attended only by learners, and do not strictly entail residency. Seminars scheduled for 1992 included:

Geometric and metaphoric models in science and
  religion/mythology
The schooner "Ernestina" adventure: An educational,
  therapeutic, and social phenomenon (focusing on "the value
  of adventure")
Yosemite and the Sierra Club: The wilderness world of John
  Muir
Mothers and daughters: Narratives of self-invention
Creativity and coenoscopy: Your approach to everything
Storytelling: A healing art

The description of the seminar titled "Geometric and Metaphoric Models in Science and Mythology" is particularly revealing. "Visual models and religious/philosophical themes," it states, "are becoming more important for scientific and humanistic research." The conveners seek to "produce a synthesis of past and present 'mytho-science.'" Their presentations "will cover several models used in quantum physics, sociobiology, and geometry." Planned activities include paired walking, brief hikes, singing, chanting, music-making, and star-charting.

Combined with the school's accreditation, the graduate program's flexibility—the opportunity to orchestrate a scholarly endeavor and wrestle with it entirely outside classrooms—appealed to me. Before attending an entry colloquium, I received no information on the subject matter of any of the seminars; an introductory booklet states simply that the graduate school faculty offers nearly forty seminars annually "on interdisciplinary topics of general interest."

I applied to The Union Institute's graduate school in March 1992. The person assigned as my advisor during the application process was Isobel Contento, Ph.D., chairperson of the department of nutrition education at Columbia University's Teachers College in New York City. Admitting a conflict of interest, she recommended that I apply to Teachers College. Despite several subsequent attempts to reach her by mail and through her answering device, I received no further communication from her.

After my acceptance as a "new learner," I briefly attended an entry colloquium held at Tufts University in July 1992. Political correctness was the order of the day. Several of the eighteen other learners had earned master's degrees through nontraditional, short-residency programs. We were a motley crew, with backgrounds ranging from "Art/Anthropology," "Art/Theology," and psychoanalysis to marketing and international relations. During the first day, several participants made public their advocacy of theism and/or vitalism. They were not challenged. One learner was a Unitarian minister and another was a former theology major. The latter, an avowed theist aware of my atheistic leanings, expressed his conviction that I could not develop a purely descriptive, unbiased doctoral manuscript on the therapeutic manifestations of the vital-force hypothesis.

The institute's "Blue Book," appropriately described as formidable by a faculty member, was distributed on the first day. It is a large, blue loose-leaf binder containing reams of information on policies, procedures, seminars, and faculty, including guidelines for preparing the doctoral transcript. The book foreshadows what learners will have mastered upon completion of the program: paperwork management and a dubious societal agenda. Prospective applicants whose interest is sparked by a desire to bypass the rigorous red tape ordinarily encountered in the pursuit of a doctorate are apt to be disappointed by the lengthy rigmarole sweetened with lofty jargon. I certainly was.

The following day, I conversed at some length with Fontaine Maury Belford, Ph.D., the institute's immediate past-dean. Fontaine "specializes" in eight different fields, including philosophy and religion, comparative mythology, futurism, and comedy. She referred to Gary Null as "that crazy nutritionist." Having read my preliminary doctoral program proposal, she expressed fascination with the subject matter, but stated that a descriptive work on the various manifestations of the "vital principle" was untenable because the principle was inextricable from the "spiritual" systems enclosing it. My approach was, in a word, unholistic.

There was much affirmative talk of holism and a paradigm shift, and we were encouraged to "extend" ourselves by selecting seminars having little or nothing to do with our academic aims. Fontaine recommended a seminar entitled "Comedy and Tragedy." The co-conveners evidently placed a premium on tolerance and diplomacy. One spoke approvingly of acupuncture and "complementary" medicine. But two learners privately voiced to me their discontent with the religious mood of the colloquium.

Is The Union Institute the "New Age" equivalent of a bible college? I consider science and religion not only incompatible but mutually destructive. Religion seems to have the upper hand at The Union Institute, and both program flexibility and "interdisciplinarity" are apparently taken to extremes that leave the significance of its degrees open to question. I withdrew from the program while the entry colloquium was in progress, and eventually received a partial refund.

Hallowed Halls of Learning?

Since early 1989, I have accumulated brochures and bulletins from many sources of dubious healthcare-related credentials. Some of these credentials can be obtained simply by paying a fee; others require completion of coursework. Some are available through correspondence courses, some entail attendance at seminars, and others involve months or years of classroom attendance. Educational standards in the United States are set by a network of accrediting agencies approved by the U.S. Secretary of Education or the Council on Postsecondary Accreditation. Accreditation is not based on the soundness of academic content, but on such factors as record-keeping, physical assets, financial status, make-up of the governing body, catalog characteristics, nondiscrimination policy, and self-evaluation system. Some of the schools described below have achieved accreditation,

Academy of Natural Healing at the Harrison Health Institute
  New York City
The academy offers training in reflexology, acupressure, nutrition, herbology, juice therapy, creative visualization, aromatherapy, polarity energy balancing, emotional healing, homeopathy, color therapy, "and much more!" Programs cover diagnosis of food allergies, a supplement for preventing PMS depression, vitamins for preventing memory loss, appetite-suppressant herbs, "a substance made by bees that dramatically increases your sexual vigor," and "easy-to-prepare teas that flush out your liver and quell cravings for alcohol and addictive drugs." A three-month series of classes leads to certification. The flyer I received from the school in late 1992 states: "Graduates of our programs are considered by many as the 'elite' of Health Consultants. . . . The demand for qualified stand-out-in-the-crowd Natural Healing Consultants grows by the day."

American Association of Nutritional Consultants, Las Vegas, Nevada
This organization is not an educational enterprise, but "a professional association dedicated to maintaining ethical standards in nutritional and dietary consulting." Apparently, the only membership requirements are submission of one's name and address and payment of a $50 fee. This

"professional member" certificate, adorned with gold seal and red ribbon, was issued in 1985 to a pet hamster:

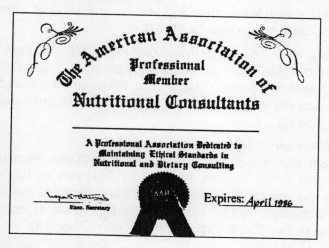

(The hamster's name, which was inscribed in calligraphy, has been deleted in order to protect its identity.)

American College of Nutripathy, Scottsdale, Arizona
This unaccredited correspondence school offers courses leading to certificates in "nutripathy," a pseudoscience that employs urine/saliva analysis as a diagnostic tool (see Chapter 12).

American Health Sciences Institute, Manchaca, Texas
This institute, operated by T.C. Fry, is "affiliated" with Health Excellence Systems and offers the same course in Natural Hygiene (see Chapter 4).

American Holistic College of Nutrition, Birmingham, Alabama
This correspondence school offers two programs leading to a "Ph.D." degree in nutrition. Its president, Lloyd E. Clayton, Jr., N.D., also operates the Clayton School of Natural Healing, which has the same address. Required doctoral courses include herbology and homeopathy. American's handsome 1992 bulletin states: "Those in the field of Health Food Store Management will find much to help them in the nutritional aspects of their business."

American Institute of Holistic Theology, Youngstown, Ohio
The postcard I received states: "The Doctor of Divinity Program from the American Institute of Theology can teach you how to practice as a

professional health teacher under the Constitutional guarantee of freedom of religion. The course provides a holistic approach to health based on fundamental principles of Nutrition and Natural Healing found in the Bible." Tuition is approximately $1,200.

Atlantic Academy of Classical Homeopathy (AACH), New York City
AACH offers a 500-hour "classroom study program. . . culminating in a Certificate in Homeopathy (C.Hom.)." In 1991, tuition was $1,500. The certificate was previously designated "Certificate in Homeopathic Therapeutics" ("CHT").

Atlantic University, Virginia Beach, Virginia
This school shares facilities and personnel with the Association for Research and Enlightenment, operated by followers of Edgar Cayce. Although it is unaccredited, it awards an M.A. degree in "transpersonal studies," a term described in its catalog as "an appropriate expression of the philosophies of the Edgar Cayce tradition" (see Chapter 4).

Bastyr College, Seattle, Washington
Bastyr is the only accredited naturopathic school in the United States. Its offerings include degrees in naturopathy and Oriental medicine (see Chapter 4). It also provides training materials for "health food" retailers through a program sponsored by the National Nutritional Foods Association. In the January 1993 issue of *Health Foods Business*, a Bastyr representative stated that the program for retailers can help employees "give intelligent and correct answers to general questions such as 'How do homeopathic remedies work?' and 'What herbs will help me to rest?'"

Bernadean University, Van Nuys, California
A division of the "Church of Universology," this correspondence school has operated without authorization in Nevada and California. Bernadean's "College of Health Sciences" has offered a "Doctor of Naturopathy" (N.D.) program, and programs leading to the titles "Certified Herbalist," "Certified Dietitian," "Certified Homeopath," "Certified Iridologist," and "Alternative Cancer Specialist."

Biological Immunity Research Institute, Scottsdale, Arizona
This institute, North American University, and the American College of Nutripathy have the same address (see Chapter 12).

BioSonics Institute, New York City
The institute's courses and classes include Aura Balancing, Pendulum, Distance Healing & Spiritual Cleansing, BioSonic Mantric Dream Repatterning, and BioSonic Tuning Fork Repatterning,

Boulder Graduate School (BGS), Boulder, Colorado
BGS offers M.A. degree programs in psychology and counseling and in health and wellness. Courses include "Sufi Psychology: A Path to the Heart," "Symbolic Aspects of Personal Growth: Astrology," and "Holistic Nursing."

California Coast University, Santa Ana, California
Formerly California Western University, this correspondence school offers a "Ph.D." program in psychology.

California College for Health Sciences, National City, California
Accredited by the Home Study Council (not a regional accrediting agency), this correspondence school offers, through its "Center for Degree Studies," an M.S. program in community health administration and wellness promotion. Students have the opportunity to "challenge" and thus bypass any course by submitting a summary of prior learning and completing a final exam or project.

California Institute of Integral Studies, San Francisco
This accredited school offers a Ph.D. program in "East-West" psychology and certification in "Integral Health Studies." Courses in the latter program cover the "energetics" of nutrition, herbal medicine, "life energies East and West," acupressure, shiatsu, shamanism, and ritual healing. According to its mission statement, one of the school's objectives is "the integration of the religious, mythic and symbolic philosophies of ancient traditions with the empirical, analytic paradigms of modern science."

California School of Herbal Studies, Forestville, California
This school offers a certificate course in "therapeutic herbalism" by correspondence, "designed to lay solid foundations for the skilled use of herbal medicines." According to its brochure, the course may be utilized "as the corner stone of developing a practice as a medical herbalist."

Chicago National College of Naprapathy, Chicago, Illinois
This school offers a three-year program leading to the "Doctor of Naprapathy" (D.N.) degree. According to its 1987–89 catalog: "Naprapathy relies primarily on specific connective tissue manipulative therapy to relieve neurovascular interference, which may generate circulatory congestion and nerve irritation. Naprapathy contends that once this interference is reduced, the body's homeostatic mechanisms will tend to return to their optimal levels of function." The curriculum includes three nutrition courses. Practitioners are not licensed (see Chapter 12).

Clayton School of Natural Healing, Birmingham, Alabama
This correspondence school offers programs leading to "Doctor of Naturopathy" ("N.D."), "Doctor of Holistic Health" ("H.H.D.") and "Doctor of Science" ("D.Sc.") degrees. Its president also operates the American Holistic College of Nutrition, which has the same address. Its N.D. program includes courses in herbology, nutrition, acupressure, reflexology, iridology, homeopathy, and "theories of cancer, diet and fasting."

Clayton University, St. Louis, Missouri
This correspondence school has offered doctorates through a Nutritional Science Institute and two other "institutes." It has awarded credits for "life experience" as well as for credits earned previously at other schools. The form letter I received stated: "If you enroll before September 15, we will send you at no cost a lapel pin with the Clayton University logo in gold—a $40 value." When I called in November 1992, a recorded message informed me that the school was neither mailing catalogs nor admitting students from the United States "at this time." Transcripts were proffered at $20 apiece.

Coast University, Honolulu, Hawaii
Formerly Gold Coast University, this degree mill offered a nonspecific "doctoral program" costing $2,695 before it was closed by federal authorities in 1992. Before the end, however, the school had a half-price "tuition" sale.

College of Health Science, Austin, Texas
This was T.C. Fry's prototypal Natural Hygiene school (see Chapter 3).

Colorado Herbal Institute (CHI), Boulder, Colorado
CHI offers residential certification programs in comparative herbology, traditional Chinese herbology, Western herbology, and Ayurvedic and yoga therapy.

Columbia Pacific University, San Rafael, California
This school bills itself as "the largest non-resident graduate university in the United States." Its School of Health and Human Services offers "Ph.D." and "D.Sc." programs in health services administration, health sciences, and wholistic health sciences. According to its brochure, credit is awarded for "prior academic work, independent study, and other relevant educational experiences."

Dominion Herbal College, Burnaby, British Columbia, Canada
This correspondence school awards the titles "Chartered Herbalist" and "Master Herbalist" to those who successfully complete the respective programs. Its president is a chiropractor.

Dr. Jay Scherer's Academy of Natural Healing, Santa Fe, New Mexico
"Accredited" by the "Career College Association" (not a regional accrediting agency), this nonprofit educational organization was founded in 1979 by Dr. Jay Scherer (1907-1990), a naturopath. Scherer was introduced to "natural healing" by his mother, a graduate of the Rudolf Steiner School in Germany (see Chapter 8). The academy offers a program leading to certification as a massage therapist. Core-program courses cover applied kinesiology, diet, homeopathic theory and first aid, hydrotherapy, naturopathic use of herbs and folk remedies, reflexology, Touch for Health, and the integration of spiritual ideals with financial goals. Continuing education courses include basic herbology and shiatsu, the latter covering *ki*, the "meridian systems," the "chakra systems," and the "five element" theory. A supplement to the catalog describes a course in "Life Impressions Bodywork"—"a healing process combining soft tissue restructuring, subtle fluid balancing, principles of Ayurvedic Medicine, and the techniques of Hakomi body-centered psychotherapy." Under the heading "Philosophy," the brochure states: "We are spirit. . . . We create and shape our physical form, using consciousness and the basic five elements." The purpose of Life Impressions Bodywork is "to 'update' our idea-imprinted tissues, releasing our bound beliefs, limitations, and energy."

Emperor's College of Traditional Oriental Medicine
Santa Monica, California
Emperor's College offers a "Master of Traditional Oriental Medicine" program leading to what its bulletin describes as "a professional graduate degree."

Foundation for Shamanic Studies, Norwalk, Connecticut
This is "a non-profit incorporated educational organization" that touts itself as "the world's leading organization devoted to the preservation, study, and teaching of shamanism." The term "shamanism" refers to a variety of magico-religious systems purported to manipulate good and evil spirits. The foundation offers "advanced workshops and training courses" in "Shamanic Extraction Healing" and "Soul Retrieval," which are "designed exclusively for people who want to bring shamanic healing work into their practice with others." The course schedule states: "Before enrolling . . . please make sure that you have been having success in contacting your power animals and/or teachers on your own." An introductory letter states that the foundation has "an active health research program which includes the study of the impact of shamanic drumming and journeying on health and on the immune system."

Harmony College of Applied Science, Los Altos, California
This "religious" correspondence school sent me three primitive, typewritten course catalogs. It offers a "master course of natural nutrition," a program leading to a "Doctor of Psychology degree," and, through the "International Society of Naturopathy" (at the same address), "doctoral" programs in naturopathy and homeopathy. Harmony awards credits for "life experience" as well as for credits previously earned at other schools.

Harold J. Reilly School of Massotherapy, Virginia Beach, Virginia
The Reilly School operates under the auspices of Atlantic University. It offers a 600-hour diploma program in massage therapy, which includes instruction in shiatsu, foot reflexology, hydrotherapy, diet, and preventive healthcare based on the "psychic readings" of Edgar Cayce (see Chapter 5).

Healing Tao Center, Huntington, New York
Courses include "Chi Kung" ("energy mastering exercise"); "Taoist Five Element Nutrition"; "Healing Light Kung Fu"; and "Lesser," "Greater," and "Greatest Enlightenment."

Health Excellence Systems, Manchaca, Texas
This is another of T.C. Fry's enterprises (see Chapter 4).

Heartwood Institute, Garberville, California
According to an introductory letter, Heartwood's "wholistic approach to health combines techniques and concepts to deal with the total human being: mind, body, and spirit." Its residential "healing arts" programs, all unaccredited, include a nine-month, 750-hour massage therapist program, a 700-hour "transformational therapist" program, an addiction counselor program, and three-month training programs in polarity therapy, Zen shiatsu, acupressure, and hypnotherapy. The massage therapist program is said to be approved for certification by the American Massage Therapy Association (AMTA) Commission on Massage Therapy Accreditation/ Approval. Electives in this program include "Jin Shin Jyutsu Self-Help" and "Creating Our Reality." Other courses include Craniosacral Technique for Practitioners; Healing with Whole Foods; Hydrotherapy; Hypnotherapeutic Bodywork, an "intensive" for those "who are interested in releasing buried emotions and memories that may be causing chronic pain, injury and illness"; and Horticultural Therapy, which "builds on the observation that many people find peace and release from stress in the garden." An "intensive" called "Nutrition for the 90's: A Practical Integrative Approach" is described as "a comprehensive, non-dogmatic approach to nutrition education aimed at improving the quality of life and health

service. . . . The demand for nutritional health educators is increasing dramatically. This training responds to the need for sensitive and sensible nutrition educators."

Himalayan International Institute of Yoga Science and Philosophy Honesdale, Pennsylvania

Until 1992, the institute offered a two-year, four-semester, residential "graduate-level" Program in Holistic Studies. Previously called the Program in Eastern Studies and Comparative Psychology, it focused on "Eastern and contemporary psychology, Eastern philosophy, holistic health, and research methodologies." According to the institute's Summer 1991 program guide: "Opportunities exist to apply study in this program to a master's or doctoral degree, as part of a pre-defined plan of independent study, through cross-registration with selected degree-granting institutions. Faculty members are available to provide guidance in formulating and applying for such independent study programs." Such opportunities existed at Lesley College in Cambridge, Massachusetts, which offers an independent study program leading to master's degrees, and at Goddard College and Norwich University, both in Vermont. However, an institute receptionist informed me in December 1992 that the Program in Holistic Studies is no longer available as such and is "not accredited anymore."

The institute scheduled a "Healing Force Series" of six seminars for "health practitioners" for 1993. Seminars center on nutrition as "a foundation for holistic treatment," homeopathy as a "catalyst for self-transformation," *prana* and "energy medicine," Ayurveda, and other subjects. Those who attend all six seminars will receive a certificate of completion. The seminar brochure states: "This training will prepare one to work in a multidisciplinary clinic and to deal effectively with the integration of a wide variety of therapeutic approaches." (See Chapter 6).

Institute of Chinese Herbology, Oakland, California

The institute offers correspondence and residential programs leading to certification as an herbalist. Its brochure states that continuing education credits are available for nurses.

Institute of Health Sciences, San Diego, California

This school offers residential programs leading to certifications, which include: massage technician, shiatsu technician, clinical massage therapist, nutritional counselor, hypnotherapist, chiropractic assistant, fitness consultant, and holistic health practitioner. The institute's "nutritional counselor" program includes a course in herbology. Its 1989–90 catalog states that "Energetic Touch" is taught at the school. This method is said to produce "a parasympathetic nervous system state known as the experience of *Zen*."

Institute of Transpersonal Psychology, Palo Alto, California
This school offers correspondence programs leading to a certificate in transpersonal or spiritual studies, a correspondence program leading to an "M.A." degree in transpersonal psychology, and a "Ph.D" degree program in transpersonal psychology. Pamphlets define transpersonal psychology as "the extension of psychological studies into consciousness, spiritual growth, body-mind relationships, and personal transformation. . . . It assumes that spiritual levels and awareness are genuine." The "M.A." program includes courses in Judaic, yogic, and Sufi perspectives on psychology, Christian mysticism, Zen Buddhism, bodywork, hatha yoga, and Jin Shin Do, described as "a system of acupressure designed to balance energies, release tension, and align the individual spirit with universal spirit."

Integral Yoga Institute, New York City
The institute has offered courses covering "food combining," *pranayama*, chanting for children, spiritual and health-enhancing skills for persons with AIDS, and "karma yoga" ("selfless service"), and workshops on "muscle-testing" for food allergies, the relationship between yoga postures and "meridians" ("energy pathways"), imagery and healing, body/mind psychotherapy, diet and nutrition, and "food laws for staying well and the secret to a balanced diet through proper acid-alkaline proportions." It also offers a yoga teacher training course.

International Correspondence Schools (ICS), Scranton, Pennsylvania
A subsidiary of the National Education Corporation, ICS bills itself as "The World's Leader in Home-Study Training." It shares its address with North American Correspondence Schools and the Center for Degree Studies. Its School of Fitness and Nutrition offers a diploma course for aspiring "nutrition counselors," "professional fitness trainers," and "exercise professionals." There are no prerequisites for this course, which ordinarily costs $699 and can be completed in less than a year. An introductory letter states that the student will learn "how to alleviate depression, level mood swings, and much more." William Shatner ("Captain Kirk" of "Star Trek") has been a television spokesperson for ICS.

International Foundation for Homeopathy (IFH), Seattle, Washington
Founded in 1978, IFH is a membership organization for health professionals and laypersons. Its activities include: (1) seminars, conferences, and

training programs; (2) a bimonthly newsletter; (3) public education; and (4) support for homeopathic research. IFH's long-term goals include establishment of a homeopathic medical school. Its educational offerings have included a five-week, 180-hour "postgraduate course in classical homeopathy for professionals" and a 126-hour course in Advanced Acute Homeopathy, "designed to meet the needs of non-medically trained people who desire comprehensive homeopathic training." The latter course is claimed to "enable students to treat acute illnesses and first aid situations."

International Institute of Holistic Sciences, Glendale, Arizona
The American College of Nutripathy referred to this "institute" in its 1989 curriculum guide. It has no telephone listing anywhere in Arizona, and it is not listed in recent editions of *Bear's Guide* (see Chapter 12).

International Institute of Theology, Glendale, Arizona
This institute became Westbrook University (see below). It was listed in the eleventh edition of *Bear's Guide,* but its phone number was disconnected as of December 1992, and there is no listing for the school in the Glendale/Phoenix area. According to a booklet published in 1989 and priced at $5, institute programs included a residential program in "pastoral hypnotherapy"; a "Ph.D." program in "cognitive sciences," with courses such as "Anesthesia and Pain Management," "Client Centered Therapies," and "Metaphysical Use of Mind Energy"; and home study courses applicable to "degree" programs, such as "Psycho Therapeutic Concepts," "Clinical Applications," "Healing Through the Power of the Mind," "Applied Mind Energy," "Psychic Development," "Esoteric Healing," "Telepathy and the Etheric Vehicle," "A Treatise on White Magic," "The Science of Alternative Healing," and "Treatment or Scientific Prayer."

John F. Kennedy University, Orinda, California
This accredited school offered M.A. degree programs in "transpersonal psychology" and "holistic health education." According to its catalog, transpersonal psychology "expands psychology to include the spiritual aspects of human experience." All of its programs have been discontinued except an M.A. program in career development.

Keys Institute, Key Largo, Florida
A 1992–93 mailing describes this institute as a nonprofit, nondenominational "human potential center" that offers retreat workshops on a small private island. It was founded in 1987 by its director, Dorothy N. Thomas, M.A., on a "simple yet solid spiritual healing base which is committed to awareness and acceptance of WHAT IS." Workshops subjects include

Native American Medicine, "holotropic breathwork," past-life therapy, and "psychonavigation" ("shamanic journeying").

Kushi Institute, Becket, Massachusetts
This is the mecca of macrobiotic educational activities (see Chapter 3).

Lafayette University, Aurora, Colorado
The American College of Nutripathy referred to this "university" in its 1992 curriculum guide. It may be defunct. (See Chapter 12.)

LaSalle University, Mandeville, Louisiana
This correspondence school offers "doctoral" and other programs through the education ministry of the World Christian Church. "Doctoral" areas of specialization include health services management. LaSalle also offers a "Certified Holistic Practitioner (CHP)" program.

Lewis Harrison Institute, New York City
In 1991, the institute offered three "holistic certification" programs in "natural healing," including a ten-month "Certified Health Consultant" program. According to a flyer, all classes covered reflexology, nutrition, herbs, "natural food preparation," and "emotional healing skills." It is now called the Harrison Health Institute (see "Academy of Natural Healing," above).

Life Science Institute, Manchaca, Texas
This was a Natural Hygiene correspondence school operated by T.C. Fry (see Chapter 4).

Loving Touch Center of New York, New York City
The center offers a two-day Reiki training seminar. A mailing states that Reiki means "Universal Life Energy." However, "Reiki is not a religion and does not require a belief system to work."

Maharishi International Institute of Vedic Science
  Cambridge, Massachusetts
The 1991-92 catalog of this unaccredited school offered three "M.S." degree programs: in Vedic science, Vedic science teaching, and Ayurveda (see Chapter 6).

Maharishi International University (MIU), Fairfield, Iowa
MIU was founded in 1971 by the Maharishi Mahesh Yogi. The next year, it began offering nondegree educational programs in Santa Barbara, California. Not long afterwards, Parsons College in Fairfield, Iowa, went broke and was purchased by the Maharishi. In 1974, MIU moved from

Santa Barbara to the 262-acre Fairfield campus. Enrollment dropped by 75 percent. In 1978, according to James Randi in *Flim-Flam!*, an MIU assistant professor of physics described the MIU campus as free of all tensions and learning difficulties "because all students had direct access to cosmic consciousness, the source of *everything*." In 1980, MIU became accredited. The Summer 1991 *TM-EX Newsletter* states that MIU "holds the Iowa state record for cumulative default rates on federally insured student loans." (See Chapter 6).

Naropa Institute, Boulder, Colorado
This accredited, supposedly "nonsectarian" college offers an M.A. degree program in "contemplative psychotherapy." According to its 1988-90 catalog, this program draws "largely on the 2500-year-old contemplative tradition of Buddhism" and "does not provide a broad background in current psychological theory."

National College of Naturopathic Medicine, Portland, Oregon
National College is not accredited, but is a "Candidate for Accreditation" with the Council on Naturopathic Medical Education, which is officially recognized by the U.S. Secretary of Education and a few states (see Chapter 4).

National Institute of Nutritional Education (NINE), Aurora, Colorado
NINE is a nonprofit corporation launched in 1980 by the National Nutritional Foods Association, a health-food industry trade organization, to provide training and credentials for "health food" retailers. It dispenses the designation "Certified Nutritionist" (CN) to those who complete a correspondence course in "nutrition counseling" and pass a written examination. NINE's 1992 catalog states that the designation is "far more than a title; it is a precise definition of a person's competence, experience and intelligence in the complex profession of nutrition counseling." The catalog claims that students will be prepared to support the premise that "diet and diet supplementation can help many problems usually treated with drugs and surgery." Ads in *East West Natural Health* call NINE "The Leader in Nutritional Education" and list nine reasons to enroll: knowledge of nutrition, counseling skills, professional enrichment, credibility, expertise, certification, independent study, continuing education, and "your opportunity in this growing field." The "Philosophy" section of NINE's catalog states: "While we in the United States may be one of the best fed people in history, we are also one of the most malnourished." Some of the "textbooks" used in the CN course are books written for the general public

that advocate treatment methods with no scientific basis. An article in the January 1993 issue of *Health Foods Business* states that NINE has awarded the CN designation to about 735 people (at least half of whom are affiliated with health-food stores) and has "educated" an additional seven thousand.

Natural Gourmet Institute for Food and Health, New York City
This enterprise was founded in 1977 by Annemarie Colbin, who writes in *Food and Healing* (1986): "It seems to me a reasonable probability that we derive nourishment not only from the macro- and micro-nutrients in foods, but from their energy fields as well. . . . The subtle energy of foodstuffs (bioenergy, force fields, chi, ki, prana, name it what you will) nourishes our own energy field." The school offers a "Food and Healing Intensive," which covers "the Chinese Five-Phase Theory and its relevance to balanced health, moods and menu planning." The Winter 1993 class schedule states that this course includes a discussion of "how to use the pharmacy in your kitchen to heal headaches, fevers, colds, skin problems, digestive disorders and other health problems. . . . It is for anyone interested in a low-tech or soft medicine that empowers people to take care of their own health on a daily basis." The school also offers a six-session course in "Healing Techniques," and courses and classes dealing with AIDS and nutrition, Ayurveda, Chinese herbology, "cooking to heal Candida," macrobiotics, and "nutrition and metabolic typing."

Nature's Sunshine Products' Distributor School
Nature's Sunshine Products' Natural Health and Business School
  Spanish Fork, Utah
These are two-day courses designed to train distributors who sell Nature's Sunshine products (see Chapter 11).

Newport University, Newport Beach, California.
Originally named Newport International University, this correspondence school offers programs leading to a "Doctor of Psychology" degree and a "Ph.D." degree in human behavior. A form letter invites the prospective student to "*JOIN THOSE SELECTED FEW* who have earned the *RIGHTS* and *PRIVILEGES* which accompany the possession of a valid *UNIVERSITY DEGREE*." In 1991, the school mailed me a "half price offer."

New York Actualism Center, New York City
The center offers a training program in actualism, described in a brochure as "training in the use of energy tools and techniques of 'inner light fire,' in which light illuminates the darkened areas of consciousness, and consuming fires eliminate the conditions that obstruct awareness and separate us from ourselves and others."

New York Open Center, New York City
This "holistic learning center" offers courses in acupressure, Anthroposophy, *A Course in Miracles,* craniosacral therapy, foot reflexology, herbalism, "holotropic breathwork," homeopathy, *I Ching, ki* breathing, kundalini awakening, meditation, past-life therapy, psychic self-defense, the psychology of the chakras, sacred dance, shamanism, shiatsu, synchronicity, therapeutic touch, Taoist healing, the tarot, yoga for weight loss, etc.

New York Training Institute for NLP, New York City
Founded in 1979, the institute conducts certification programs in neurolinguistic programming (NLP; see Glossary) and in Ericksonian hypnosis. It has also offered various workshops, such as "Evolution's End," which explored "the profound biological dynamic between the heart and mind."

North American University, Scottsdale, Arizona
This "university" shares offices with the American College of Nutripathy (see Chapter 12).

Nutritionists Institute of America, Inc., Kansas City, Missouri
This correspondence school offers a three-month "Assistant Nutritionist" course, a six-month "Associate Nutritionist" course, and a twelve-month "Nutritional Consultant" course, all leading to "certification." In 1984, the *Kansas City Star* described how one of its reporters had secured a diploma from the institute in the name of a pet dog. The dog's final grade average was said to be in the "upper 2 percentile range" even though the reporter had deliberately submitted many wrong answers in preliminary tests and had not returned one of the eight pages of the final exam.

Nyingma Institute, Berkeley, California
The institute offers a "Kum Nye" teacher training program leading to conferral of a Teacher Training Certificate. Its catalog describes "Kum Nye relaxation" as a set of tension-relieving exercises based on Tibetan medicine and Buddhist "body-mind" disciplines. The catalog also states that the institute is licensed by the State of California Board of Registered Nursing as a continuing education provider for registered nurses.

Nyingma Institute of Colorado, Boulder, Colorado
This institute was an affiliate of the Nyingma Institute in Berkeley, California, which offers a certification program in human development based on Tibetan Buddhism. The Colorado facility's Winter 1991 course schedule included a course in "Kum Nye"—a stress management method that supposedly "can penetrate the ordinary physical, emotional and

mental constrictions to natural energy flow." The schedule stated that the course was approved as a continuing education activity by the Colorado Nurses' Association and that the Association was accredited by the American Nurses' Association Board of Accreditation. But by December 1992, there was no Nyingma Institute in Colorado.

Ohashi Institute, New York City
This "nonprofit educational and cultural organization" offers a program by which one can become a "Certified Ohashiatsu Instructor or Consultant." A course schedule defines Ohashiatsu as "Wataru Ohashi's method of balancing life energy in the body." According to the schedule, Ohashiatsu can "rejuvenate body, mind, spirit."

Omega Institute for Holistic Studies, Rhinebeck, New York
Omega describes itself as "a holistic education center at the forefront of personal and professional development in a variety of subject areas, from health and psychology to multicultural arts and spirituality." The center offers courses on ancient dowsing techniques, "chakra power animals," dream interpretation, "dreamwork," "holistic nursing," homeopathy, meditation, out-of-body experiences, "psychospiritual counseling," and yoga. The core workshop in its wellness program covers diet and nutrition.

Polarity Education Center of New York (also called Polarity Wellness Center, Inc.), New York City
According to a flyer, the center's "courses and certification programs are in alignment with and fulfill national Polarity Therapy standards for practice." The flyer further states: "By tuning into natural currents of life energy we can learn how to heal ourselves and others." Courses include Advanced Cranial Balancing, Digestive & Elimination Anatomy, Dream Counseling, Relationship Counseling, and Polarity Business Practices.

Rolf Institute, Boulder, Colorado
This institute offers Rolfing training at various locations, leading to certification. According to its flyer, Rolfing, or "structural integration," is a "pioneering form of bodywork and movement education," a unique approach to manipulating muscles and connective tissues that can relieve pain and stress, change body structure, and "benefit people in psychotherapy by facilitating a deeper connection to their emotional conflicts." The institute's basic training program can take one to two years to complete and costs between $10,000 and $12,000. Its supplemental reading list includes *Craniosacral Therapy, Experience of No Self*, M. Scott Peck's *The Road Less Traveled, and* Fritjof Capra's *The Turning Point*.

Rosemont College, Rosemont, Pennsylvania
Rosemont is an accredited liberal-arts college with several majors. In addition, however, it offers a Health Perspectives Program of instruction in a variety of "alternative" methods. The 1993 offerings include a course in Ayurveda, which spans three weekends and costs $1,050. Taught by a naturopath, it "provides enough of the essentials . . . to help participants integrate this experience into their personal and professional lives," but is "not for diagnosis or treatment for oneself and others."

Rudolf Steiner College, Fair Oaks, California
This unaccredited school's three full-time programs include an introductory program covering such topics as "Parsifal and the Quest for the Holy Grail," a teacher-education program, and an arts program, which "can lead to pedagogical or therapeutic application." (See Chapter 8).

Sarasota School of Natural Healing Arts, Sarasota, Florida
Sarasota offers a Professional Massage Therapy Training Program, which includes courses in nutrition, pet massage, and polarity therapy, and a course called "AIDS 101." Another, "advanced" program covers "the concepts of Chi as the vital life force," the "five element theory," and the "energetic" functions of organs.

Satchidananda Ashram-Yogaville, Buckingham, Virginia
This ashram (religious community residence) offers teacher training programs in yoga and meditation leading to "certifying" diplomas. Instruction is provided in nutrition and how to teach the practice of "pure diet."

School of Classical Chinese Herbology, New York City
The school offers a full-time, two-year diploma program.

School of Healing Arts, San Diego, California
Begun in 1984 as the Institute of Health Sciences, this nonprofit school offers a Massage Technician certification program, which covers "parasympathetic massage," shiatsu, and "energy balancing"; a Shiatsu Technician certification program, which includes courses in Oriental health assessment and traditional home remedies; a Nutritional Counselor certification program, which includes courses in herbology, "comparative nutritional systems," basic first aid, and legal and ethical aspects of business practices; a Clinical Massage Therapist certification program, which includes courses in hydrotherapy and "Body Psychology & Counseling"; and a Clinical Hypnotherapist certification program. The school also offers courses in "Zen-Touch Body Balancing," which cover Ayur-

vedic principles, "constellational influences," "energy and life force concepts," macrobiotics, and yin/yang "polarity effects."

School of Natural Healing, Springville, Utah

Founded in 1953 by the late herbalist John R. Christopher, N.D., this school offers an "Herbal Diploma" program via correspondence, and a "Master of Herbology Diploma" program, which requires attendance for ten days and the writing of a 5,000-word "master's thesis." A 1993 flyer lauds Christopher as a "lone stalwart" who, "although relentlessly persecuted by orthodox medicine," maintained a keen sense of humor and dedicated the last years of his life to spreading the "herbal word." An earlier flyer offered a "Doctor of Herbology" program.

School of Spiritual Science, Medical Section, Fair Oaks, California

This school was established by occultist Rudolf Steiner in 1923, in Dornach, Switzerland, to be the "esoteric core" of the General Anthroposophical Society. It is open only to members of the Anthroposophical Society of America. Its medical section includes physicians, nurses, pharmacists, art therapists, and massage therapists. Other Anthroposophical "initiatives" include the Anthroposophical Nurses Association of America and the Physicians' Association for Anthroposophical Medicine, both in Kimberton, Pennsylvania, and the Anthroposophical Therapy and Hygiene Association in Spring Valley, New York (see Chapter 8).

Southwest University, New Orleans (Metairie), Louisiana

This correspondence school offers "Ph.D." programs in counseling psychology, holistic health sciences, and hospital/health services administration.

University of Bridgeport, Bridgeport, Connecticut

This accredited university offers a program with weekend attendance that leads to an M.S. degree in human nutrition. This program's faculty includes a chiropractor certified by the American Chiropractic Board of Nutrition, and a registered dietitian who promotes unscientific nutrition practices and is pursuing a doctorate through The Union Institute. (In 1985, the American Dietetic Association censured this dietitian for failing to adhere to accepted standards of practice.) The university opened a chiropractic college in 1990. Plagued by serious financial problems, however, it was purchased in 1992 by an affiliate of Reverend Moon's Unification Church.

Vega Study Center, Oroville, California

Founded by Herman Aihara, this center serves under the auspices of the George Ohsawa Macrobiotic Foundation. (See Chapter 3.)

Waldorf Institute of Sunbridge College, Chestnut Ridge, New York
This Anthroposophical institute offers two "M.S.Ed." degree programs in
Waldorf education, both of which, according to its bulletin, are "accredited" by the State of New York Board of Regents (not a regional accrediting
agency). It also offers an evening program that includes courses in doll-
making, eurythmy, "form drawing" ("a therapeutic artistic activity"), and
"ensouled speech." (See Chapter 8.)

Westbrook University, Phoenix, Arizona
Westbrook was formerly the International Institute of Theology. Its phone
number was not in service in November 1992, and there was no listing for
the school in the Phoenix area. Encompassing four "colleges," including
the College of Holistic Sciences, Westbrook offered a "Ph.D" degree, a
"Doctor of Divine Metaphysics" ("MeD.D.") degree, and others.

Attacking the "Opposition"

To bolster their own credibility, individuals with dubious credentials often
attack those with respectable credentials. For example, in *Eat to Succeed*
(1986), "Dr." Robert Haas claims (incorrectly):

> The basic difference between a registered dietitian . . . and a
> nutritionist with a master's or doctoral degree in nutrition is that
> the non-R.D. nutritionist often is better educated in biological,
> biochemical, and nutritional sciences than the registered dietitian.
> In my opinion, minimal training often fails to provide the practi-
> tioner with enough nutritional and scientific background to pre-
> scribe diets and nutritional supplements for people with acute
> nutritional problems.

Haas, identified on the book's jacket as a "clinical nutritionist," says
he holds a doctorate from "an international university recognized by the
British and Canadian governments." Actually, his "Ph.D." degree came
from an unaccredited correspondence school.

What's Out There?

What is the net result of this crazy quilt of credentials? I believe it is harmful
"health care" and the entrenchment of ignorance.

In September 1992, as a member of the National Council Against
Health Fraud's Task Force on Diploma Mills, I telephoned all businesses

listed under the headings "Nutritionists" and "Dietitians" in the 1992-93 NYNEX Yellow Pages for New York City's Borough of Queens. Only one of the twenty-six businesses listed appeared to be a reliable source of nutrition information, and at least seven were "health food" stores or supplement distributors. Three GNC stores were listed under the heading "Dietitians."

My phone calls yielded some interesting responses. A self-styled "certified eating-disorder specialist" told me he prescribes supplements. When I specified tiredness as my chief complaint, he declared that tiredness is "the first sign of illness." A "holistic nutrition" practitioner also said he prescribes supplements and stated he holds an N.D. (Doctor of Naturopathy) degree "from Puerto Rico." When I asked where I could buy the supplements, he responded that he had a "warehouse" in his office.

As my favorite former professor, Dr. John Orta, tells his students, "Everybody who eats thinks he's a nutritionist."

The Bottom Line

The health marketplace is flooded with both pretenders to scientific nutrition and patently vitalistic "nutritionists." Some are sincere but misguided, while others are obvious charlatans. Their activities are not limited to preaching to the gullible. They spread cultism in the guise of science, and crusade to undermine public confidence in science itself. Many oppose established public health measures such as fluoridation, food irradiation, immunization, and even the pasteurization of milk. The harm they do has not been measured, but certainly is not small.

Susan V. Greene, R.D., a dietitian from Cincinnati, Ohio, has noted that American consumers fall prey to misleading nutrition claims because they lack the "big picture" concerning food and diet. In a letter in the January 1993 *Journal of the American Dietetic Association*, she said:

> If all Americans could learn, starting in elementary school, about food—its properties; how to use it in a balanced menu; how to buy it; . . . how it relates to chronic disease or chronic good health; and *really* learn how to practice and apply these skills like they learn how to read, write, and add—they would be less gullible when it comes to false or misleading nutrition claims. They would not attribute magical, mystical, or lifesaving qualities to individual foods or nutrients.

Glossary

Accreditation, academic: Certification that a school (or a department within a school) meets standards established by a recognized accrediting agency. Colleges and professional schools are accredited by agencies approved by the U.S. Secretary of Education or the Council on Postsecondary Accreditation.

Actualism: Process "designed to reveal the 'Actual Design' of evolving life forms and to train students to experience their untapped potential for creative self-expression and joyful communication with all forms of life," according to the New York Actualism Center (see Chapter 15). It was developed in the 1950s by Russell Schofield, a theistic clairvoyant with doctorates in psychology, naturopathy, and divinity. Both of Schofield's parents had been ordained ministers.

Acupressure: Generic term encompassing all forms of massage involving the stimulation of acupuncture points (see below). Acupressure systems include shiatsu (see below), Do-in (Oriental self-massage, as taught at the Kushi Institute), acu-yoga (a series of yogic postures and stretches), and *Tui Na* (Chinese massage).

Acupuncture: A system of treatment purported to balance the body's "life force," usually by inserting needles into the skin at points where imaginary horizontal and vertical lines ("meridians") meet on the surface of the body. These points are said to represent various internal organs (some of which are nonexistent). Although acupuncture can sometimes relieve pain, there is no evidence that it can influence the course of any organic disease.

Alexander technique: Process of posture improvement through maintenance of an alignment of the head, neck, and back, which is supposed to lead to optimum overall physical functioning. Proponents claim that it is useful in the treatment of a variety of diseases, including asthma, hypertension, peptic ulcer disease, and ulcerative colitis. Developed at the turn of the century by an Australian Shakespearean actor, Frederick Matthias Alexander (1869-1955), it is popular with performing artists. Although its original purpose was to assist voice projection, Alexander concluded that faulty posture was responsible for diverse symptoms. He postulated that habitual unbalanced movement affects the functioning of the entire body, implying that postures have consequent behavior patterns and that bad postural habits can distort one's personality. Alexander further postulated that there was one basic movement, which he termed the "primary control," from which all proper bodily movements flowed. Teachers of the technique convey it by manipulating various parts of the student's body and simultaneously repeating key phrases. One teacher has distributed a flyer titled "Bone Meditation," which states: "By separating the bones from one another, you can feel energy flow through and out the finger tips."

Alimentary canal: The digestive tract, which extends from the mouth to the anus.

"Alternative" health care: Umbrella term for a multitude of unscientific health-related practices (see Chapter 2).

A.L.S.: Abbreviation for amyotrophic lateral sclerosis (also called Lou Gehrig's disease), a fatal, progressive degeneration of the spinal cord.

Anabolism: The constructive phase of physiological processes, characterized by the conversion of substances into body components.

Anthroposophical medicine: An ill-defined pseudomedical system based on the occult philosophy of Rudolf Steiner (see Chapter 8).

Antioxidant: Any substance that in small amounts can inhibit the oxidation (molecular "degradation") of compounds in the body or in food.

Applied kinesiology: An elaborate vitalistic system of diagnosis and treatment centering on "muscle-testing." Applied kinesiology originated as a diagnostic method in the mid-1960s with Michigan chiropractor George Goodheart, who theorized that muscle groups share "energy pathways" with internal organs and that, therefore, every organ dysfunction is discoverable in a related muscle. Testing muscles for relative strength and tone supposedly taps the body's "innate intelligence" and enables practitioners to detect specific dysfunctions.

Arnold Ehret's "mucusless" diet healing system: System involving diet, fasting, eugenics, exercise, sunbaths, enemas, and bathing, developed by Prof. Arnold Ehret, a German-born Christian naturopath who died in 1922. The system is set forth in his book of twenty-five lessons, *Mucusless Diet Healing System: A Scientific Method of Eating Your Way to Health.* Ehret wrote therein: "The *Mucusless Diet* consists of all kinds of raw and cooked fruits, starchless vegetables, and cooked or raw, mostly green-leaf vegetables. The *Mucusless Diet Healing System* is a combination of individually advised long or short fasts, with progressively changing menus of *non-Mucus-Forming Foods. This Diet Alone Can Heal Every Case of 'Disease'* [even] without fasting." Citing *Genesis*, Ehret proclaimed fruits and leafy, green vegetables the "natural food of man." Most other foods, according to him, are "mucus formers"—"wrong foods" that "contain, produce and encumber the human body with the matter of disease." Ehret claimed that rice-eating was the "foundational cause" of leprosy and that "masturbation, night emissions, prostitution, etc., are all eliminated from the sex life of anyone living on a mucusless diet after their body has become clean and powerful."

Aromatherapy: The "medical" use of essential (volatile, aromatic, and flammable) oils from plants, flowers, and some wood resins. In aromatherapy, the oils are sniffed, ingested, or applied to the skin, usually via massage. Proponents claim that it can relieve hundreds of diseases and conditions. *The Aquarian Guide to the New Age* (1990) notes that "the ancient classifications of curative scents has [sic] largely been lost and New Age practice of aromatherapy is somewhat different from its traditional roots."

Asclepius (also spelled "Aesculapius" and "Asklepios"): In Greek mythology, Apollo's son, one of the chief gods of healing, around whom developed a trendsetting medical cult in ancient Greece. The temples of Asclepius functioned as sanatoria and as training centers for priest-physicians. The regimen at these temples emphasized ritual, fresh air, light, appropriate diet, hydrotherapy, massage, enemas, and topical remedies. However, they did not constitute the cradle of Greek medical science and practice, as had been generally supposed in the early twentieth century. Rather, Greek medicine derived from the observations of early philosophers and gymnasium trainers. Hippocrates, for example, said that "sacred" diseases—diseases supposedly inflicted by the gods—had a natural cause and appeared to him "nowise more divine nor more sacred" than other diseases. (See Chapter 4.)

Aston patterning: Method for affecting the emotions through manipulation of the body, developed by Judith Aston in collaboration with Dr. Ida Rolf, the originator of Rolfing (see below).

Astral body: In Theosophy (see below), the imperceptible, semimaterial "model" or "framework around which the physical body develops, a vehicle for *prana* ("life-energy") that survives the death of the physical body.

Atherosclerosis: Accumulation of deposits of cholesterol and fibrous tissue within the inner walls of large and medium-sized arteries.

Aura: In the world of the occult, an envelope or "spiritual skin" of "subtle energy" that surrounds magnets, crystals, and the living bodies of humans, animals, and plants. Supposedly visible to clairvoyants, human auras are said to reveal the passions and vices of the soul.

Aurasomatherapy: Method of diagnosis and treatment concocted by British "clairvoyant" Vicky Wall, aimed at revitalizing and "rebalancing" the body's supposed "aura." It involves color, herbal extracts, and essential oils.

Auricular reflexology: Form of reflexology (see below) focused on the ear, "discovered" in 1967 by Dr. Nogier of France.

Auriculotherapy: A variant of acupuncture based on the notion that a set of points on the outer ear represents a fetus (with its head near the earlobe) and that these points correspond to body parts. Proponents claim that illness can be diagnosed by examining the ear for tenderness or variations in electrical conductivity, and can be relieved by acupuncturing that part of the ear "corresponding" to the anatomical source of the malady.

Autism: A severe developmental disorder characterized by lack of interest in and responsiveness to others.

Autogenics (autogenic training and autogenic therapy): System of "self-hypnosis" involving various methods, including "affirmations," biofeedback, meditation, regular breathing, repetitive utterances, "stream-of-consciousness" vocalizations, visualization, and baroque music. Biofeedback is the technique of using monitoring devices to furnish information on autonomic (automatic) bodily functions—such as heartbeat, blood pressure, and temperature—in an attempt to gain some voluntary control over them. The term "autogenics" was coined by German psychiatrist and neurologist Johannes H. Schultz, who developed its principles and methods in the 1920s and 1930s. Its premise is that the body will balance itself naturally when it is directed into a state of relaxation, a state that promotes self-discovery and enhances awareness. Proponents claim that autogenics is useful in the treatment of alcoholism, allergies, asthma, diabetes mellitus, diarrhea, hypertension, indigestion, migraines, premature ejaculation, sinus tachycardia, and ulcers. However, they report a side effect, "autogenic discharge," which has a variety of manifestations, including tearing of the eyes, muscle spasms, jerking of the limbs, and a sensation of floating.

Ayurveda (Vedic medicine): The traditional Hindu system of medicine, a form of naturopathy. (See Chapter 6.)

Behavioral kinesiology: A variant of applied kinesiology (see above) developed by psychiatrist John Diamond, M.D., and described in his book *Behavioral Kinesiology* (1979). *Applied Kinesiology* (1987), by Tom and Carole Valentine, cites Diamond's definition: "an integration of psychiatry, psychosomatic medicine, kinesiology, preventive medicine and the humanities."

Bioenergetics (bioenergetic analysis and therapy): Popular offshoot of a psychoanalytic theory developed by Wilhelm Reich (1897–1957), an associate of Sigmund Freud and the "discoverer" of a (nonexistent) "primordial cosmic energy"—which he called orgone—released with sexual orgasm (see "Orgonomy," below). Bioenergetic therapy is a sometimes painful, "psychotherapeutic" form of bodywork (see below) developed by Alexander Lowen (1910–), a psychiatrist. According to bioenergetics, the human body is an "energy system," energy must flow freely for health to be maintained, and all body cells record emotional or "energetic" reactions. These cellular "memories" supposedly can be used for healing or consciousness-raising. The patient is said to release them by screaming, crying, and kicking.

Bioflavonoid: Pigmented substance, not essential in humans, once thought to have vitamin activity. There is no scientific evidence that bioflavonoids are useful in the treatment of any human ailment.

BioSonics: Sound therapy involving music, tuning forks, crystals, massage, astrology, "color breathing," and mantras.

Bodywork: "New Age" umbrella term for modalities that involve manipulation and/or exercise of the body and, usually, supposed alignment of its "energy field" or removal of blockages to the flow of "energy." Examples are acupuncture, the Alexander technique, bioenergetic therapy (see above), chiropractic manipulation, reflexology, Reiki, Rolfing, seiki-jutsu, and therapeutic touch (see below).

Cachexia: A condition of wasting illness and malnutrition.

Chakra: Derivative of the Sanskrit word *cakram,* meaning "wheel" or "circle." It refers principally to an indefinite but large number of alleged spherical loci of the body that collect *prana,* the "life force" (see Chapter 3). Chakras are said to be visible only to clairvoyants. According to Theosophy (see Chapter 8), they are the sense organs of the "etheric double," a supposed invisible replica of the physical body that functions as a conductor of "vitality." Three of the chakras are said to be utilized only in black magic.

Chelation therapy: A series of intravenous administrations of a synthetic amino acid (EDTA) plus various other substances. Proponents claim, without substantiation, that it can reverse atherosclerosis and is useful against many other diseases.

Chiropractic: A pseudoscientific system devised in 1895 by Daniel David Palmer, an Iowa grocer and fish seller who believed that a vital force— which he termed the "Innate"—expressed itself through the nervous system. Some chiropractors still cling to this belief, some reject it completely, and some consider spinal problems an "underlying" cause of disease. (See "Subluxation," below, and Chapter 14.)

Christian Science: An antiscientific system of religious ideas, "discovered" by Mary Baker Eddy (1824-1910), which contends that mind is the only reality and that illness, pain, and death are the results of "wrong thinking" (see Chapter 2).

Clairvoyance: Alleged ability to directly perceive things (such as remote objects or future events) that are impossible to perceive via the human senses alone.

Colon: Large intestine. Many vitalists incorrectly regard the colon as a "toxic waste dump" that necessitates such modalities as colonic enemas and "internal cleansing" products to "detoxify" the body.

Color therapy (chromotherapy): Treatment involving light, food, clothing, and environment, based on the belief that colors have wide-ranging curative effects. "Color therapists" claim that cures result from correction of "color imbalances." Many hold that the seven colors of the spectrum correspond to the seven major chakras ("energy centers" of the body). Modern color therapy is based partly on the teachings of two mystics who were interested in "auric" colors: Rudolf Steiner and Charles W. Leadbeater (see Chapter 8). The means of diagnosis and treatment vary from practitioner to practitioner.

Complementary medicine: Medical practice said to integrate established (scientific) and "alternative" health-care methods (see Chapter 7).

A Course in Miracles: Best-selling, Christian-oriented self-study course, first published in 1975, around which a metaphysical movement has developed. It was supposedly authored by Jesus Christ, courtesy of his channel, Helen Schucman (1909–1981), a research psychologist at Columbia University. Schucman expressed bafflement over the book's alleged source, but her father had owned a metaphysical bookstore during her childhood. (See Chapter 2.)

Craniosacral therapy (cranial technique, cranial osteopathy, or craniopathy): Supposed manipulation of skull bones (which, in fact, are fused to one other and not "adjustable") into alignment in order to remove impediments to a patient's "energy." The "therapist" holds the skull in his hand and supposedly attunes himself to the patient's "rhythm." Proponents claim that about 95 percent of all people suffer from misalignment of cranial bones, which, they say, causes toothaches, migraines, and neurological disturbances.

Creative visualization: "Healing" system of positive thinking and imaging developed by "New Age" spiritual teacher Shakti Gawain (1947–). Gawain defines creative visualization in her bestseller of the same name: "the technique of using your imagination to create what you want in your life." She further defines imagination as "the basic creative energy of the universe."

Cult: Any unscientific system that encourages obsessive devotion to a person or an ideal.

Discharge: In macrobiotics, the elimination of toxins from the body via urination, defecation, coughing, sneezing, cysts, tumors, and other mechanisms.

Dreamwork: Systematic inquiry into or use of dreams for healing and self-development.

Dualism: This term has several meanings. Broadly, it refers to any philosophical doctrine asserting the existence of natural and supernatural realms, matter and spirit, body and soul, and good and evil. Plato and René Descartes were dualists, but more modern philosophers, influenced by scientific discoveries, have tended toward monism, which holds that reality has a single ultimate nature. (See Chapter 2.)

Emetic: Substance that induces vomiting.

Empiricism: The view that experience, especially of the senses, is the best source of knowledge.

Endodontist: A dentist specializing in diseases of the tooth root, the enamel pulp, and surrounding tissues.

Ethnopharmacology: The study of lore and customs relating to medications.

Exorcism: Alleged expulsion of evil spirits.

Extentional medicine: A seldom-used term for "complementary" medicine (see above).

Five elements: Term based on two Chinese words, *wu* ("five") and *xing* ("move" or "walk"), whose implicit meaning is "five processes." According to ancient Chinese tradition, earth, metal, water, wood, and fire are the five manifestations ("phases" or "transformations") of *Ch'i* or *Qi* ("life energy"), of which all things are composed. In Chinese medicine, each "element" is a symbol for a category of related functions and qualities: "earth" represents balance or neutrality; "metal," a period of decline; "water," a state of maximum rest leading to a change of functional direction; "wood," a growth phase; and "fire," maximum activity.

Flower essence therapy: "Therapeutic" use of liquid "extracts" from flowering plants. Preparation of the "extract" involves immersion of a flower in water and subsequent exposure of the liquid to sunlight or heat, whereby it supposedly becomes imbued with healing "life energy" and "spiritual elements" from the flower. Intuition and "muscle-testing" are two means by which flower "remedies" are selected.

Food combining: Any dietary practice based on the incorrect notion that various combinations of foods consumed during a meal can cause or correct illness.

Gift of tongues (speaking in tongues): Uttering words (usually foreign) and/or making meaningless or unintelligible vocal sounds in a state of religious ecstasy. Christian theology considers this a gift of the Holy Spirit.

Hair analysis: A test in which a small quantity of hair, usually from the nape of the neck, is analyzed for its mineral content. Hair analysis has limited usefulness as a screening test for poisoning by lead or other heavy metals. However, it is not valid for determining nutritional status.

Herbal medicine: "Medicine" based on herbal traditions, which, according to Michael McIntyre in *Herbal Medicine for Everyone* (1988), "emphasize the indivisibility and interaction of mind and body, matter and spirit."

High-colonic enema (colonic irrigation): An alleged "detoxification" method typically performed by pumping twenty or more gallons of warm water (sometimes with herbs or coffee added) intermittently into and out of the lower gastrointestinal tract through a rubber tube inserted twenty to thirty inches into the rectum.

Hinduism. A complex of sociocultural and religious beliefs and practices that elaborated in the region of India and Pakistan. Hinduism features: (1) yoga (see below); (2) a system of hereditary classes (castes); (3) the view that all forms ("essential natures") and theories are aspects of a unique external being (pantheism); and (4) belief in nonviolence (*ahimsa*), karma (the total of ethical consequences), caste duty (*dharma*); reincarnation (passing of the alleged soul into a new human body or another life-form), and nirvana (see below).

Holistic medicine: Treatment of the "whole person." The term "holistic" is often used to promote many types of unscientific practices whose stated goal is to integrate body, mind, and "spirit" (see Chapter 2).

Hologram: A three-dimensional photographic image.

Holotropic therapy (holotropic breath therapy or holotropic breathwork): A psychotherapeutic technique developed in the 1970s by psychiatrist Stanislav Grof, M.D., and his wife, Christina. Holotropic therapy involves breathing exercises, sound technology (including music), physical therapy, and the drawing of mandalas—aids to meditation symbolizing the unity of the soul with the universe. One of the goals of holotropic therapy is to produce mystical states of awareness by releasing emotional conditions frozen in tissues.

Homeopathy: An unsubstantiated, vitalistic system of "energy medicine" developed by German physician Samuel Christian Hahnemann (1755–1843). Homeopaths treat diseases with minute doses of substances—or with their alleged nonphysical, "quintessential" forms. According to homeopathy, the most effective remedy for a particular disease is that which can produce in a healthy person all the symptoms of the disease if a substantial amount is administered. In *Homeopathy: Medicine of the New Man* (1979), teacher and practitioner George Vithoulkas states that one proof of the existence of the "vital force" is "the fact that when the disturbed organism of a patient is properly tuned through the administration of the right homeopathic remedy, the patient not only experiences the alleviation of symptoms, but also has the feeling that life once again is harmoniously flowing through him." He further writes that homeopathy "actually bases its entire system upon the stimulation of that force." (See Chapter 11.)

Hydropathy ("water cure"): Internal and external use of water as a near-panacea (see Chapter 4).

Hydroponics: The cultivation of plants in a mineral solution rather than in soil.

Hydrotherapy: The use of water to treat disease. In scientific medicine, hydrotherapy is a mode of physical therapy in which water is used externally. Unscientific hydrotherapy includes both internal and external uses of water.

Hygeia: The ancient Greek goddess of health, daughter of Asklepios (Asclepius), the god of medicine. Asklepios was originally a legendary physician; he attained mythological godhood during the fifth century B.C.E. It has been said that Hygeia and Asklepios represent poles of medical thought: Hygeia, a lifestyle-oriented approach based on "natural laws"; Asklepios, a skeptical, disease-oriented approach.

I Ching **(Book of Changes):** Term combining two Mandarin words meaning "divination" (*Yi*) and "classic" or "book" (*Jing*). The *I Ching* is a Chinese book of ancient origin that is consulted as an oracle, or tool of divination. It is part of the canon of Confucianism, the quasi-religious philosophy that dominated China until the early twentieth century.

Incarnation: Religious concept referring to the period of time one spends in a particular body.

Interactionalism (mind/body interactionism): An unscientific, dualistic theory that regards mind and body as separate and distinct realities (see Chapter 2).

Iridology: A pseudoscience according to which the functional state of body components can be appraised by examination of the iris (the colored portion of the eye surrounding the pupil). Proponents hold that the iris serves as a map of the body and that warning signs of physical, mental, and spiritual problems can be found there. The modern version of iridology is ascribed to Dr. Ignatz von Peczely, a Hungarian who discovered the supposed "iris-body" connection in his childhood, when he broke the leg of an owl and a black stripe spontaneously appeared on the owl's iris.

Jin shin (or *jin shin jyutsu*): Translated as "the art of circulation awakening," jin shin is a form of shiatsu (see below) instituted by Jiro Murai. It is performed on patients in a meditative state, and involves only the thirty major bilateral acupuncture points, and gentle, prolonged "point-holding."

Kahuna healing: General term for the "therapeutic" practices of kahunas—traditional Hawaiian medicine men (shamans). Huna—which literally means "that which is hidden, or not obvious"—is the native philosophy of the Hawaiian Islands. Its current emphasis is on healing and ESP. The literal meaning of kahuna is "keeper of the secret." Kahunas are priestly practitioners of magic who supposedly are capable of foretelling the future and reviving the dead. They are believed to be conduits for *mana*, the "life force," which can be controlled through breathing and visualization exercises.

Karma: Literally, "deed." In Hinduism, Buddhism, and other Oriental religions, karma is the total effect of an individual's actions over all of his or her incarnations (see above).

Ki: Japanese word signifying both breath and attention ("mental force"). It refers to an alleged original, fundamental, supernatural, governable, creative "energy of being" concentrated in the abdomen.

Kirlian diagnosis (aura analysis): Method whereby characteristics of a person's "aura" (an alleged, normally invisible "energy field" or "bioplasmic body") are recorded via Kirlian photography. "Auric" qualities are alleged to reveal variations in health and emotional state. Kirlian photography was developed by Soviet electrician Semyon Kirlian and his wife Valentina in the late 1950s. This process does not involve a lens, but placement of an object upon unexposed film atop a metal photographic plate, and the addition of an electrical field. Kirlian patterns have been correlated with acupuncture meridians, but Kirlian diagnosis has been debunked by scientists who found that such physiological variations at the surface of the skin as moisture, temperature, and pressure account for the differences in the "auras."

Kundalini: Sanskrit term essentially meaning "coiled." It is often referred to as the "serpent power," for it is likened to a snake coiled at the base of the spine. Yogis and other paranormalists believe that kundalini is ordinarily dormant, primordial cosmic energy, which can be activated by *pranayama* (see below) and other yogic practices; depending upon one's skill and wisdom, activation results in enlightenment or in madness, malignant disease, or enfeeblement.

Leukocytosis: An abnormal increase in the number of white blood cells (leukocytes) in the blood, generally caused by infection.

Live-cell analysis: Diagnostic method whereby a patient's blood is examined via a dark-field microscope with a television monitor attached. It was developed by James Privitera, M.D., a Californian who had been convicted of conspiracy to distribute laetrile as a cancer cure, sentenced to six months in jail, and pardoned by then-Governor Jerry Brown. Proponents claim that live-cell analysis can reveal many health problems, represented by "abnormalities" visible on the monitor, that are treatable with food supplements.

Macrobiotics: A multifaceted, diet-centered, Eastern oriented, metaphyscial movement founded by George Ohsawa (see Chapter 3).

Mea culpa: Latin expression meaning "through my fault"; an acknowledgment of personal guilt or error.

Medical astrology (astrologic medicine): Diagnostic, prognostic, and therapeutic practice based on the notion that correspondence exists between specific mental and physical conditions and the relative positions of celestial bodies.

Meditation: The act or process of giving continuous undivided attention to something.

Meridians: Hypothetical channels through which the body's "life force" is said to circulate.

Mesmerism: Theory and practice of proto-hypnotic "animal magnetism" or "mind healing" based on the career of Franz (or Friedrich) Antoine Mesmer (1734–1815), a flamboyant Viennese physician who had originally planned to become a cleric. Mesmer theorized that an invisible, magnetic fluid permeates the universe, connecting human beings with one another and with the stars, and that disease was the result of inadequate supplies of this fluid. According to Mesmer, the task of the true doctor was to restore the equilibrium of the vital fluid among people. This he sought to accomplish with magnets, musical instruments, and tubs of water containing iron filings. Mesmerism was first debunked formally in 1784.

Metaphysical: Concerning the nature of reality (being, the universe).

Mysticism: The doctrine or belief that knowledge of God, spiritual truth, ultimate reality, and other matters said to defy intellectual understanding is obtainable by subjective means independent of reasoning and the five senses.

Naprapathy: A variant of chiropractic based on the philosophy that contractions of the body's soft tissues cause illness by interfering with neurovascular function. Proponents claim that gentle stretching of ligaments, muscles, and other connective tissues of the spine and joints can restore health by relieving such interference. Naprapathic practice also includes nutritional, postural, and exercise counseling. Practitioners are not licensed.

Narcolepsy: Disorder characterized by recurrent, uncontrollable, brief episodes of sleep.

Natural Hygiene: Spartan form of naturopathy that emphasizes fasting and food combining (see Chapter 4). Hygienists eschew pharmaceutical products, herbal remedies, nutrient supplements, and foods derived from animals.

Natural laws: A term used by advocates of "alternative" medicine to connote a morality of nature and to support various notions that modern eating habits and other behavior cause diseases unknown to primitive peoples. In *Health at the Crossroads: Exploring the Conflict Between Natural Healing and Conventional Medicine* (1988), Dean Black, Ph.D., former president of two health-food companies, writes: "There is some higher principle that must first be honored. . . . *Nature has its own laws and may not allow intrusion without revenge.* . . . Our only choice is to seek a way of getting along with nature that doesn't pit us against her, that instead allies us with her, capturing her strength for our own."

"Nature": In "alternative" healthcare, a salutary, creative, guiding force; a synonym for "vital force" (see below) or God.

Naturopathy (naturopathic medicine): A variegated system—vitalistic, lifestyle-oriented, and supposedly "drugless"—whose basic theory is that disease results from the violation of "natural laws" (see "Natural laws," above, and Chapter 4). Naturopaths claim to cure by strengthening the body's "vital force."

Necrotic tissue: Dead tissue.

Neologism: Newly coined term.

Neurolinguistic programming NLP): Behavior-modification technique based on an alleged reciprocal relationship between physiology and vocal tone, posture, and eye movements. It was initially formulated in 1975 by Richard Bandler and John Grinder, who reputedly duplicated the "magical results" of several top communicators and therapists, including Milton H. Erickson, M.D., the originator of Ericksonian hypnotherapy. According to the New York Training Institute for NLP, NLP has six basic assumptions: (1) the meaning of your communication is the response you get, independent of your intention; (2) there is a positive intention beneath every behavior; (3) there is no failure, only feedback; (4) the map is not the territory; (5) people make the best choice available to them; and (6) all people have the resources needed to accomplish what they really want.

"New Age": A broad, amorphous, medico-religious social movement whose central characteristic seems to be a nontraditional, personal, makeshift or adjustable spirituality. In *Confronting the New Age* (1988), evangelist Douglas Groothuis, M.A., writes that this spirituality "is a rather eclectic grab bag of Eastern mysticism, Western occultism, neopaganism, and human potential psychology."

Nirvana: Complete detachment from the material world, attainable only via the extinction of individuality. In the *Occult Glossary: A Compendium of Oriental and Theosophical Terms* (1972), G. de Purucker argued that nirvana does not mean "entitative annihilation," but rather the annihilation of man's "lower principles" only and the absorption of what remains into the "Higher Self." According to *The Dictionary of Mind and Spirit* (1991), nirvana literally means "extinguishing" and entails personal *non*survival.

Nutripathy: Quasireligious system of diagnosis and treatment involving "spiritual" analysis of urine and saliva, "food combining," (see above), lifestyle, and a multitude of "supplements." It was developed in the 1970s by Gary A. Martin, an entrepreneurial, nontraditional Christian minister, and is based on a "formula" devised by self-styled biophysicist Cary Reams (see Chapter 12).

Occult: Relating to or occupied with matters allegedly involving supernatural mechanisms or forces.

Organic farming: Cultivation of food crops supposedly without pesticides or synthetic fertilizers. Foods so grown are not necessarily more nutritious, tastier, or safer than their conventionally grown counterparts.

Orgonomy: Use of devices alleged to accumulate and direct orgone to relieve a variety of ailments, including cancer and impotence. The word "orgone" was coined by Austrian-born American psychoanalyst Wilhelm Reich (1897–1957) to refer to his hypothetical fundamental, omnipresent, life-sustaining, intelligent radiation. He is said to have believed that UFOs were spaceships powered by orgone. His last book, *Contact with Space*, recounts his efforts to save the earth from alien spacemen. In 1957, Reich was imprisoned for marketing his quack devices. He died in a federal penitentiary, but the American College of Orgonomy survives. (See "Bioenergetics," above.)

Orthomolecular medicine: Form of fringe medicine based on the dubious theory that many diseases are associated with biochemical abnormalities correctable with large doses of vitamins (megavitamin therapy) and other substances normally present in the body.

Osteopathy (osteopathic medicine): Health care system similar to that of scientific medicine, but with a slight additional emphasis on musculoskeletal problems. Osteopaths (doctors of osteopathy, or D.O.s) practice predominantly in the United States, where they are the equivalent of M.D.s. However, osteopathy was originally delineated by Dr. Andrew Taylor Still (1828-1917), who taught that the body is a "vital machine" capable of producing its own remedies for infections and other diseases when it is in "correct adjustment."

Ozone therapy: Use of an unstable form of oxygen to treat disease, especially cancer, which proponents claim is caused by a deficiency of oxygen.

Paradigm: A model or overall understanding of how something works. If a new concept doesn't fit, scientists must determine whether the new concept is flawed or the current paradigm needs adjustment. An example of a faulty paradigm is the "alternative" concept that disease is cause by disturbances of the body's "vital force."

Paranormal: Unusual and apparently not explainable (or not readily explainable) in scientific terms.

Past lives therapy (past-life therapy): A form of psychotherapy that emerged in the 1960s, based upon a belief in reincarnation and usually involving hypnotism, in which the causes of present physical and psychological problems are traced to traumatic events experienced in past lives. Problems that supposedly respond well to this "therapy" include relationship difficulties, chronic guilt, phobias, compulsions, asthma, and chronic back pain.

Pharmacopeia: Book containing an official list of medications with information on their properties, preparation, and use.

Polarity balancing (polarity therapy): Supposedly "holistic" system based primarily on Ayurvedic principles, involving massage, postures, stretching exercises, diet (usually vegetarian), and positive attitude. It is alleged to restore health by removing blockages to the flow of "vital" or "universal" energy between the so-called positive (head) and negative (feet) poles of the body. Polarity therapists regard the body as a magnet. Born in 1890, the therapy's originator, Randolph Stone, was a naturopath, chiropractor, and osteopath. He retired to live in India in 1973.

Poultice: A soft, moist, usually heated mass of various composition, applied to a sore or inflamed part of the body.

Pranayama: In yoga philosophy, the "healing breath"; breathing exercises undertaken to control *prana*, the life force, and produce an altered state of consciousness.

Primal therapy: Psychotherapeutic method developed by child psychologist Arthur Janov, author of *The Primal Scream*, that dispenses with analysis and attempts to resolve neuroses through a process of painful catharsis. Janov maintained that, to be effective, psychotherapy must uncover repressed "primal pains"—unpleasant experiences undergone not only in childhood and infancy, but even in the fetal and embryonic stages. According to Janov, these can be dispelled only if they are re-experienced and given physical expression (e.g., through screaming). "Rebirthing" is the crux of primal therapy (see below). *From Acupuncture to Yoga: Alternative Methods of Healing* (1983) states: "Primal therapies constitute the most difficult form of psychoanalysis for both analyst and patient. An estimated half of those who began practicing it have since stopped."

Psychic dentistry: Supposed spontaneous and instant healing of teeth or gums in a group setting with a psychic or "holistic" dentist present.

Psychic surgery: Alleged healing of diseased tissue, or its removal with either bare hands or common instruments, without leaving a skin wound. It is actually a sleight-of-hand procedure that involves palming and releasing a red liquid represented as "blood." Some psychic surgeons claim they operate only on the patient's "etheric body," or "perispirit."

Psychometry ("object reading"): Literally, "measure of the soul." A form of clairvoyance, psychometry is the alleged ability to divine information about people and events associated with an object merely by touching, handling, or being near to the object. Psychometry was devised and named by "psychic researcher" Dr. J.R. Buchanan, who held that every object that has ever existed and every event that has ever occurred have left their impressions in the "ether" or "astral light." Buchanan supposedly discovered that when psychometry students simply held drugs, they often exhibited the symptoms that would have resulted had they ingested the drugs, and that it was possible for some psychometrists to diagnose illness simply by holding the patient's hand.

Pulse diagnosis: In traditional Chinese medicine, the examination of the pulse to discover the condition of internal organs. Like scientific physicians, practitioners of Chinese medicine use the radial artery at the wrist. However, whereas scientific practitioners takes one pulse at either wrist to determine rate and rhythm, the latter seeks six pulses at each wrist—which supposedly correspond to twelve internal spheres of bodily function—and uses such terms as "bolstering-like," "confined," "empty," "floating," "flooding," "full," "knotted," "leather," "sinking," "slippery," "soggy," "tight," and "wiry" to describe them. A "wiry" pulse, for example, is said to indicate liver disease.

Qigong (Ch'i kung): Literally, "to work the *Qi*," or vital force. "*Gong*" is a Mandarin word pertaining to skill. (Its Cantonese equivalent is "*kung*," as in "kung fu.") Qigong is a Chinese system involving patterned breathing, posture, stylized movements, and visualization. There are three main forms of Qigong: medical Qigong, often called "acupuncture without needles," and Buddhist and Taoist Qigong, which include the Chinese martial arts.

Radiesthesia ("medical dowsing"): Literally, "perception of radiation." "Radiesthesia" is the anglicized form of a French word coined in 1927 by a priest, Alex Bouly, for the process of dowsing—a clairvoyant "art" centered on finding water, minerals, animals, missing persons, lost objects, or hidden treasure, usually with an instrument such as a pendulum or divining rod (a forked rod or tree branch, or a bent wire). The term "radiesthesia" refers both to dowsing in general and to medical dowsing— the application of dowsing to the diagnosis and treatment of disease.

Medical dowsing was pioneered by three French priests, the Abbe Alexis Mermet, the Abbe Alex Bouly, and Father Jean Jurion. Mermet developed dowsing techniques to help missionaries identify medicinal plants in foreign countries. Practitioners diagnose illness by suspending an instrument over the patient, over tissue samples or body fluids from the patient, over a photograph of the patient, or over an item of the patient's belongings, such as an article of clothing. Diagnosis is based on the movements of the instrument.

Radionics (radionic therapy or psionics): *The Arkana Dictionary of New Perspectives* (1989) cites the Radionics Association's definition: "a method of healing at a distance through the medium of an instrument or other means using the ESP faculty. In this way, a trained and competent practitioner can discover the cause of disease within any living system, be it a human being, an animal, a plant, or the soil itself. Suitable therapeutic energies can then be made available to the patient to help restore optimum health.... Basic to radionic theory and practice is the concept that man and all life forms share a common ground in that they are submerged in the electromagnetic field which, if sufficiently distorted, will ultimately result in disease." Radionics was developed earlier in this century by Albert Abrams, a San Francisco-born neurologist who surmised that different diseases are related to different radio waves emitted by various parts of the body and even by tissue samples. He claimed that diseases could be relieved with devices that emitted curative vibrations. The American Medical Association called him the "dean of gadget quacks."

Rebirthing: A form of bodywork (see above) that utilizes hyperventilation and seeks to resolve repressed attitudes and emotions that supposedly originated with prenatal and perinatal experiences. Patients are expected to reenact the birth process.

Reflexology (originally called zone therapy): A generic term that refers to the stimulation of areas under the skin—usually via massage, but sometimes via acupressure or acupuncture. Reflexology is claimed to be useful in assessing and improving the function of specific body parts. Proponents hold that all bodily organs have corresponding external "reflex points" (particularly on the feet) that can be used to enhance the flow of "energy." "Reflex points" are said to exist not only on the feet, but on the abdomen, arms, back, ears, face, hands, legs, neck, nose, scalp, tongue, and wrists. Proponents claim that reflexology can relieve asthma, constipation, migraines, sinus congestion, and diseases of the kidney, liver, and pancreas. The treatment is sometimes painful.

Reiki: Japanese word meaning "spirit energy." "Reiki" refers to a religious movement begun in the late nineteenth century by Dr. Mikao Usui, a Japanese scholar and minister. It emphasized "brushing" of the body's "aura" with the hands to transfer "universal life force energy" and thus effect healing and harmony. Different schools exist, some including visualization of secret symbols.

Rolfing (structural integration or structural processing): A quasi-"psychoanalytic," stringent deep-massage technique of "muscular realignment" promoted mainly for back and neck problems. Rolfing is also alleged to facilitate weight loss, relieve anxiety, and increase stamina and self-esteem. It was developed in New York in the 1930s by Ida P. Rolf, Ph.D. (1896–1979), a physiologist who compared the technique to "rebuilding a sagging or bulging brick wall, rather than trying to prop it up by artificial means." "Rolfers" adjust the massage when they supposedly detect areas of "energy imbalance" within the body. The standard Rolfing series consists of ten sessions. Proponents claim that one's posture reveals past traumatic experiences, and that as soon as Rolfing effects emotional and "energetic" release, the body's flow of "vital energy" is restored and the mind and body are integrated. *The Encyclopedia of Alternative Health Care* (1989) describes an incomplete session that was so painful the client had to resign his job.

Sclerology: Practice of examining the sclera (white portion of the eye) for lines, discolorations, and other markings to discover the condition of some bodily organs.

Seiki-jutsu: Japanese therapy wherein a "healer" transfers *seiki*—"universal healing energy"—to a patient via the hair whorl at the crown of the patient's head.

Serum: The fluid part of the blood that remains after removal of clotting proteins and blood cells.

Shamanism: General term for a variety of indigenous magico-religious "healing" systems. The core doctrine is that all healing involves a spirit world.

Shiatsu (acupressure): Abbreviation of a Japanese word literally meaning "finger-pressure treatment." Shiatsu is a Japanese form of therapeutic massage in which pressure is applied with the palms and four fingers of each hand to those areas of the body used in acupuncture. The goal of shiatsu to promote health by increasing the flow of *ki* in the body.

Siddhis: Sanskrit word for "perfect abilities" or "miraculous powers." These include clairvoyance, telepathy, levitation, superhuman strength, the ability to "possess" others, and the power to make oneself and objects invisible. In Hindu tradition, such abilities are either inherent in the individual or acquired through austerity, drugs, meditation, or magic. The true yogi desires the siddhis not for their utility, but for their mystical significance. They are thus regarded as byproducts of training and as obstacles to be surmounted in the quest for *samadhi* (mystical ecstasy or "superconsciousness"). The highest form of *samadhi* is nirvana (see above and Chapter 6).

Subliminal tapes: "Self-help" audiotapes alleged to influence persons via the subconscious. Studies have shown that many tapes do not contain any signal that could *possibly* effect subconscious perception. Regardless, the notion is unfounded.

Subluxation: In scientific medicine, this term refers to partial dislocation of a bone, usually a vertebra. Many chiropractors use the term to represent spinal problems they claim to treat, but they do not agree among themselves on a definition. Some claim that subluxations are "bones out of place" that can "pinch" spinal nerves. Others describe subluxations as "functional impairments" of the spinal joints.

Supernaturalistic: Relating to an alleged world above and beyond the natural world of mind and matter, or to the belief therein.

Tarot: Pack of playing cards (usually twenty-two, but sometimes seventy-eight) used in fortunetelling. The tarot consists of a joker and cards depicting vices, virtues, and "elemental forces." According to *Mysteries of Mind, Space and Time: The Unexplained* (1992), "Ideally, to make consulting the Tarot a true divinatory method, each practitioner should decide exactly what meaning to attach to each card—even if this departs widely from what is commonly held to be the meaning."

Theism: Broadly, belief in the existence of one, several, or many gods; belief that the universe constitutes God; or any system based on such a belief.

Theosophy: Nonstandard, Eastern-oriented religion pieced together by clairvoyant H.P. Blavatsky (1831-1891); the forerunner of Anthroposophy (see above and Chapter 8).

Theotherapy: Method developed by author Peter Lemesurier whereby a person determines, more or less unconsciously, which Greek god or goddess best symbolizes his or her disease, and then treats the disease by trying to adopt those godly characteristics he or she considers both positive and sustainable. According to theotherapy, every such characteristic is a therapy, and every symptom of every disease is a healing tool.

Therapeutic touch: Method developed by a clairvoyant meditation teacher and a nursing professor in which the hands are said to transfer "excess energy" from practitioner to patient. It is alleged to relieve or eradicate pain and to accelerate healing.

Toning: Use of the voice to promote healing, creativity, and vitality via physical, emotional, and spiritual "attunement." Toning is said to be a means of activating the dormant "creative energy" in everyone, of "letting the body speak," and of bringing new "life energy" to "inhibited" or "unbalanced" parts of the body. It is sometimes performed with meditation.

Trance channeling: "Mediumship"; purported communication by a disembodied entity through a living person in a trance.

Urine therapy: "Remedy" with Indian roots involving topical application of urine, ingestion of urine, urine enemas, and/or urine injections. Hindus credit urine with "purifying powers" and regard urine from cows as a "sacred cleanser." In the 1970s, a former Indian prime minister stated on national television in the United States that he drank some of his own urine daily for health maintenance. He called urine "the water of life." Contemporary Western proponents of urine therapy claim it can cure acne, AIDS, arthritis, chronic fatigue syndrome, herpes, and leprosy.

Vegan: A vegetarian who consumes no meat, fish, eggs, milk, or other foods derived from the animal kingdom.

Vital force: An alleged form of energy distinct from the physical forces explainable by the laws of physics and chemistry. It is also called life force, universal life force, cosmic life force, life energy, universal life energy, vital energy, vital element, and vital principle. It has dozens of specific appellations as well, including: animal magnetism (as in mesmerism), astral light (Theosophy), "bioenergy" (Eastern Europe), *Ch'i* or *Qi* (Chinese cosmology), ether (alchemy), etheric formative force (Anthroposophy), the Holy Spirit or Holy Ghost (Roman Catholicism), *ki* (Japanese rendering of *"Ch'i"*), *mana* (Polynesia), manitou or manitu (Algonquin religion), orgone (Reichian theory), and *prana* (Hinduism). Many "alternative" practitioners claim that their methods work by manipulating such a force. (See Chapter 2.)

Yoga: Derivative of a Sanskrit word meaning "union" or "joining." Yoga is an ancient Indian dualistic and theistic philosophy whose goal is the liberation of the "true self" from material bonds via the silencing of the mind. It features a method of inward concentration consisting of psychosomatic practices aimed at the supreme yogic ideal of renunciation of the world. These practices include postures (*asanas*), breathing exercises (*pranayama*), and a mental exercise (*pratyahara*) designed to facilitate withdrawal from unpleasant stimuli. Supposedly, the "stainless" yogi ultimately attains oneness with God. The eight prominent schools of yoga and their foci are: *hatha yoga*—control of the physical body via postures, pranayama, and "purification" practices (*kriyas*); *laya yoga*—kundalini (see above) and the chakras; *mantra yoga*—mind control; *jnana yoga*—understanding of the laws of the universe; *bhakti yoga*—love and devotion to an ideal; *karma yoga*—selfless service, duty, and behavior control; *raja yoga,* which encompasses all of the foregoing schools; and tantric yoga (tantra)—ritual sex. "*Hatha*" means "sun and moon"; "*mantra*" means "to deliver mind"; "*jnana*" means "knowledge"; "*bhakti*" means "devotion"; "*karma*" means "deed"; "raja" means "royal"; and "tantra" derives from a word meaning "to weave" (e.g., unformed energies). In *The Religions of Man* (1986), Huston Smith wrote that *karma yoga* involves "a radical reducing diet that is designed to starve the finite personality to death." (See Chapter 6.)

Zarlen therapy: Advanced "mental healing" technique said to be useful in the treatment of brain damage, color blindness, dyslexia, varicose veins, and numerous other ailments. It was "discovered" by Jonathan Sherwood in 1984 in New Zealand. The therapy supposedly affords users access to knowledge acquired during previous incarnations. "Zarlen" is the name of Sherwood's spirit guide. According to a flyer from the Queensland Awareness Center in Queensland, Australia, "When Zarlen first made contact with Jonathan in 1984, he stated that he had not had communication with humans for over 25,000 years and that he had returned to assist with a spiritual transition which the human race was about to pass through."

Zen: Japanese rendering of a Sanskrit-derived Chinese word meaning "meditation." The term refers to Zen Buddhism, whose thrust, according to *The Aquarian Guide to the New Age* (1990) is "the shattering of the mindset, the breaking down of ritualized patterns of thought so that a more direct perception of reality may become possible. The methods used to achieve this result are both bizarre and interesting. Almost all are designed either to shock or to drive the mind into such a paradoxical state that it can no longer support itself."

Zone therapy: Generic term coined by Edwin F. Bowers, M.D. Zone therapy is a form of reflexology (see above) introduced in the United States in 1913 by Bowers's associate, William H. Fitzgerald, M.D., a specialist in diseases of the ear, nose, and throat, who divided the human body into ten zones and taught that "bioelectrical" energy flowed through these zones to "reflex points" in the hands and feet. In *Zone Therapy*, which underwent its eighteenth printing in 1989, proponents Anika Bergson and Vladimir Tuchak write:

> Too often, books on health written on the periphery of the medical profession have tended to sound like the work of quacks. . . . The truth is that, to this day, no one knows why this type of therapy works at all. . . . The fact remains that zones and meridians have not been explained to the satisfaction of science . . . . Nobody knows for sure why proper pressure below the big toe affects the spinal column at the shoulder level. . . . What works, works, and if it alleviates human suffering, we suggest that it should be practiced whether or not we understand it from the point of view of established science.

Recommended Reading

Anon. "Nutrition" against disease: A close look at a chiropractic seminar. *Nutrition Forum* 5:25–29, 1988. Reports on an undercover investigation of a company that marketed supplement concoctions illegally through chiropractors.

V. Aronson. You can't tell a nutritionist by the diploma. *FDA Consumer* 17:28–29, July/August 1983. Describes how the author obtained a "Nutritionist" certificate after taking a two-lesson course from Bernadean University, an unaccredited correspondence school that was not legally authorized to grant degrees.

S. Barrett. The American Association of Nutritional Consultants: Who and what does it represent? *Nutrition Forum* 3:49–54, 1986. Chronicles the history and activities of the American Association of Nutritional Consultants and three similar groups that offered dubious credentials and promoted unscientific practices.

_____ Commercial hair analysis: Science or scam? *Journal of the American Medical Association* 254:1041–1045, 1985. Indicates why hair analysis is not reliable for determining the body's nutritional state or prescribing dietary supplements.

_____ *Quackery by Mail.* New York: American Council on Science and Health, 1991. Comprehensive report on the mail-order health marketplace.

_____ Sunrider and the law. *Priorities*, Fall 1992, pp. 44–46. Describes the activities of a multilevel company whose herbal products were promoted with false claims.

275

S. Barrett. Chiropractors and nutrition: The "supplement underground." *Nutrition Forum* 9:25–28, 1992. Describes how nutrient concoctions are marketed illegally to chiropractors who prescribe them to patients.

K. Butler. *A Consumer's Guide to "Alternative Medicine."* Buffalo, N.Y.: Prometheus Books, 1992. Reports on the author's investigation of "alternative" health practices and promotions.

R. Deutsch. *The New Nuts Among the Berries*. Palo Alto, Calif.: Bull Publishing Co., 1977. Describes the activities, theories, and impact of prominent food faddists.

R.P. Doyle. *The Medical Wars*. New York: William Morrow and Co., 1985. A lucid analysis of the scientific method and its application to various medical controversies.

J. Dwyer. The macrobiotic diet: No cancer cure. *Nutrition Forum* 7:9–11, 1990. Describes nutritional hazards and unproven claims related to macrobiotic diets.

S. Dingott and J. Dwyer. Benefits and risks of vegetarian diets. *Nutrition Forum* 8:45–47, 1991. Describes how vegetarian eating can be very healthful if done wisely, but can be harmful if food selection is too restrictive.

J. Fried. *Vitamin Politics*. Buffalo, N.Y.: Prometheus Books, 1984. The classic investigation of megavitamin therapy and its proponents.

N. Gevitz (ed.). *Other Healers: Unorthodox Medicine in America*. Baltimore: The Johns Hopkins University Press, 1988. Provides a history of the botanical movement, water-cure movement, homeopathy, chiropractic, contemporary folk medicine, and several other unorthodox systems.

L.E. Grivetti. Nutrition past—Nutrition today: Prescientific origins of nutrition and dietetics. *Nutrition Today* 26(1):13–24, 1991; 26(4):18–29, 1991; 26(6):6–17, 1991; 27(3):13–25, 1992. A 4-part series on nutrition theories and food-related practices from ancient through modern times. Focuses on the legacies from India, China, the Mediterranean, and Hispanic regions.

V. Herbert and S. Barrett. *Vitamins and "Health" Foods: The Great American Hustle*. Philadelphia: George F. Stickley Co., 1981. An investigative exposé of the "health food" industry.

W.T. Jarvis. Recognizing today's nutrition quacks. *Nutrition & the M.D.* 11:1–2, December 1985. Describes the spurious credentials, invalid diagnostic tests, and questionable prescriptions utilized by unqualified nutritionists.

J.J. Kenney. Fit for Life: Some notes on the book and its roots. *Nutrition*

Forum 3:57–59, 1986. Analyzes misinformation in *Fit for Life* and the background of its authors.

H.M. Leach. Popular diets and anthropological myths. *New Zealand Medical Journal* 102:474–477, 1989. Challenges dietary fads claimed to be based on characteristics of traditional or primitive societies.

L. Lindner. The new, improved macrobiotic diet. *American Health* 7:71–86, May 1988. Describes macrobiotic dietary practices and the author's visit to the Kushi Institute as a patient.

J. Lowell. The Gerson Clinic. *Nutrition Forum* 3:9–12, 1986. Describes the author's first-hand investigation of the Gerson Clinic in Tijuana, Mexico.

J.G. Melton (ed.). *New Age Encyclopedia.* Detroit: Gale Research Inc., 1990. Provides more than three hundred factual accounts of the people, organizations, practices, and philosophies related to New Age activities. Describes how the New Age and holistic health movements share ideology and are intertwined.

M.E. Potter, A.F. Kaufmann, P.A. Blake, et al. Unpasteurized milk: the hazards of a health fetish. *Journal of the American Medical Association* 252:2048–2052, 1984. Debunks vitalistic claims that raw milk is superior to pasteurized milk and describes the transmission of infection posed by raw-milk products.

J. Roth: *Health Purifiers and Their Enemies.* New York: Prodist, 1977. An overview of the struggle between "natural health" advocates and the scientific community.

R. Schafer, E.A. Yetley. Social psychology of food faddism. *Journal of the American Dietetic Association* 66:129–133, 1975. Defines food faddism and discusses various ways that it may meet psychological needs.

A. Skolnick. Maharishi Ayur-Veda: Guru's marketing scheme promises the world eternal 'perfect health.' *Journal of the American Medical Association* 266:1741–1750, 1991. Criticizes some of the claims and marketing practices of Ayurvedic proponents. Letters commenting on the article were published in *JAMA* 266:1769–1774, 1991.

P. Skrabanek and L. McCormick. *Follies and Fallacies in Medicine.* Buffalo, N.Y.: Prometheus Books, 1990. Contains excellent chapter debunking "alternative medicine."

J. South. Can nutripathy transform the world? *Nutrition Forum* 4:57–61, 1987. Describes the philosophy and activities of Gary Martin and his American College of Nutripathy.

———— The Manner Seminar. *Nutrition Forum* 5:61–67, 1988. Describes the unscientific theories and practices of "metabolic therapy," as promoted by the late Dr. Harold Manner.

D. Stalker and C. Glymour (eds.). *Examining Holistic Medicine.* Buffalo, N.Y.: Prometheus Books, 1985. A devastating exposé of "holistic" propaganda and practices.

V.E. Tyler. False tenets of paraherbalism. *Nutrition Forum* 6:41–44, 1989. Debunks ten types of myths promoted by unscientific herbalists.

————— *The New Honest Herbal.* Binghamton, N.Y.: Haworth Press, 1993. A referenced evaluation of more than one hundred herbs and related substances.

G. von Nostitz et al. *Magic Muscle Pills!!: Health and Fitness Quackery in Nutritional Supplements.* New York: New York City Department of Consumer Affairs, 1992. Reports on an investigation of the "bodybuilding supplement" industry.

J. Whorton. *Crusaders for Fitness: A History of American Health Reformers.* Princeton, N.J.: Princeton University Press, 1982. Describes the life and times of many of the early promoters of food faddism and "hygienic religion."

J. Yetiv. *Popular Nutritional Practices: A Scientific Appraisal.* Toledo, Ohio: Popular Medicine Press, 1986. (Current address: P.O. Box 1212, San Carlos, CA 94070.) A referenced analysis of more than one hundred nutrition topics of current concern.

D. Zimmerman. A case report: How Pat McGrady's 'CANHELP' helps patients with cancer. *Probe* 1(2):4–7, 1991.

J.F. Zwicky, A.W. Hafner, S. Barrett, and W.T. Jarvis. *Reader's Guide to "Alternative" Health Methods.* Chicago: American Medical Association, 1993. An analysis of more than 1,000 reports on questionable approaches to solving health problems.

Index

East West Books, 6
East West Journal, 29
East West Natural Health, 29–30, 49,
   194
Eaton, Stewart C., 124
Eddy, Mary Baker, 15
Edgar Cayce Foundation, 66
Ehret, Arnold, 253
Emerson College of Herbology Ltd.,
   227–228
Emetic, 258
Emperor's College of Traditional
   Oriental Medicine, 237
Empiricism, 17–19, 258
Endodontist, 258
Enemas,
   in Ayurvedic medicine, 89
   coffee, 135–136, 140–141, 142
Enviro-Tech Products, 111
Enzymes, food, 221
Ephedrine, 201, 202
Erewhon, 29
"Ergogenic aids," 202–207
Esko, Edward, 37–38, 41–42
Esko, Wendy, 37
Eternal Life Center, 189
Ethnopharmacology, 258
Eurythymy, 119–121
Exorcism, 258
Extentional medicine, 258

FAIM; *see* Foundation for the
   Advancement of Innovative
   Medicine (FAIM)
Faithful, Marianne, 82
Farrow, Mia, 82
FDA; *see* Food and Drug
   Administration (FDA)
Federation of American Societies for
   Experimental Biology, 205–206
Ferguson, Marilyn, 15
Feuerstein, George, 12
FibreSonic, 146
Finch, Dr. Caleb, 209

Fit for Life, 53, 58, 60, 62
Fitzgerald, Dr. William H., 273
Five element model, 160, 258; *see also*
   Chinese medicine
Flower essence therapy, 258
Follies and Fallacies in Medicine, 114
Food and Drug Administration (FDA)
   enforcement actions, 28, 108, 145,
     205, 215
   and homeopathic products, 164
Food combining, 57–58, 258
Foster, Steven, 175
Foundation for Shamanic Studies, 237
Foundation for the Advancement of
   Innovative Medicine (FAIM),
   97–114, 228
   purposes of, 97–98
   symposia by, 100–112
Fredericks, Carlton, 3, 99
Free Spirit, 43
Fritz, Norman, 133
Fry, T.C., 52–56, 58
Fuller, Robert C., 47, 213

Galen, 11
General Nutrition Corporation (GNC),
   5, 250
George Ohsawa Macrobiotics
   Foundation, 30, 248
Gerber, Dr. Richard, 15
Gerovital H3, 3
Gerson, Charlotte, 133, 134–140
Gerson, Dr. Max B., 129–133, 186
Gerson Institute, 133, 139
Gerson therapy, 129–142, 226
   evaluations, 131–133, 141–142
Gerson Therapy Center, 133, 137, 138,
   139–140
Gift of tongues, 2, 258
GlanDiet, 162–163
Glucose tolerance factor, 206
Gold Coast University, 236
Goldman, Albert, 82
Goode, Tom, 148